the
FAT
smash
diet

the **FAT** *smash* *diet*

the last diet you'll ever need

Dr Ian K. Smith

Vermilion
LONDON

3 5 7 9 10 8 6 4

Copyright © Ian K. Smith 2006

First published in the United States in 2006, by St. Martin's Griffin

First published in the United Kingdom in 2007 by Vermilion,
an imprint of Ebury Publishing, Random House,
20 Vauxhall Bridge Road, London SW1V 2SA

Random House Australia (Pty) Limited
20 Alfred Street, Milsons Point, Sydney,
New South Wales 2061, Australia

Random House New Zealand Limited
18 Poland Road, Glenfield,
Auckland 10, New Zealand

Random House South Africa (Pty) Limited
Endulini, 5A Jubilee Road,
Parktown 2193, South Africa

Random House Publishers India Private Limited
301 World Trade Tower, Hotel Intercontinental Grand Complex,
Barakhamba Lane, New Delhi 110 001, India

Random House UK Group Limited Reg. No. 954009
www.randomhouse.co.uk

Papers used by Vermilion are natural, recyclable products made from wood grown in sustainable forests.

A CIP catalogue record for this book is available from the British Library

ISBN 9780091917050

Printed and bound in Great Britain by Bookmarque Ltd., Croydon, Surrey

Copies are available at special rates for bulk orders. Contact the sales development team on 020 7840 8487 or visit www.booksforpromotions.co.uk for more information.

To Lynn Cherry, my beautiful aunt,

May you lead a longer, healthier and happier life now that you're one hundred pounds lighter.

In the words of the great singer Barry White:

"I love you just the way you are."

THE FAT SMASH DIET

AUTHOR'S NOTE

Many of my American readers have either seen or heard of my diet programme on the popular VH1 show *Celebrity Fit Club*. Over the past year I have received thousands of e-mails from viewers asking me to share with them the diet that I have put many Hollywood celebrities on with tremendous success. I want to get something clear right from the beginning. This is not a 'celebrity' diet. This is a diet for EVERYONE. It is not based on gimmicks or false promises or fake science like a lot of other programmes you'll find on the market. This is a nutritionally sound, scientifically based programme that if followed correctly will deliver results even to those who have not succeeded on other diets.

With many years of experience working with tens of thousands of dieters, I have learned as much from the people who are trying to lose weight as they have learned from me. One of my biggest lessons – most dieters want a simple, easy-to-follow, realistic plan that does not require a tremendous expenditure of money or time. Dieters want to be able to eat reasonably, which means enjoying an ice cream cone or a couple of chocolate chip cookies or a slice of pizza every so often. It's ridiculous to think that people are going to go through the rest of their life without having a slice of cake for dessert or a drink of alcohol when socialising with family and friends. What I've learned is that if a meal plan includes a good percentage of 'likeable' foods, then people are much more willing to stick to that programme than they will to a programme that eliminates all of the 'fun' foods and makes unrealistic dietary demands.

I followed the advice and lessons I've got from thousands of dieters living all over the world. These pages are full of *only* relevant information, as I have – excuse the pun – trimmed the fat to give you just the essentials that you will need to be successful. I created The **FAT SMASH DIET** as an answer to all of the diet questions I've received over the years and the pleas from people who are simply fed up with being overweight. The **FAT SMASH DIET** is easy to follow, inexpensive, forgiving, and healthy. You will get as much out of it as you put into it. It has worked for not only Hollywood celebrities, but my friends and family members who couldn't believe they lost so much weight while still eating many of the foods they have always enjoyed.

You too can finally shed the weight and start feeling good about yourself both on the outside and inside. Remember, if you cheat, you're only cheating yourself. But if you follow the programme and remain dedicated, you will be transformed into a new you, ready to take advantage of all the great things that life has to offer.

Enjoy!

– Dr Ian Smith
New York City
January 2006

CHAPTER 1
The FAT SMASH DIET Philosophy

Diets don't fail people; people fail diets. The **FAT SMASH DIET** is a programme that will never fail you if you open your mind to the great possibilities, believe in yourself and give a full commitment. The **FAT SMASH DIET** is designed to be a forgiving programme that is as much about helping people make the necessary lifestyle changes to lead a healthier, happier and longer life as it is about getting rid of extra weight that only increases your odds of developing devastating medical complications such as high blood pressure, diabetes and heart disease. I'm a realist. Most people have a difficult time following diets to the letter, slipping every once in a while when they can't resist the urges or when they've reached a plateau and feel like the weight is no longer coming off. The **FAT SMASH DIET** understands this and allows you to dial back into the programme if necessary, by returning to Phase I, getting back on course then resuming the programme where you left off.

The **FAT SMASH DIET** is a 90-day programme with four phases that will ultimately re-wire your body and its relationship to food and physical activity for the rest of your life. This is not about short-term fixes that will eventually fade and put you back where you started. Instead, this is about life change for the long term! At the end of the 90 days, you will have made small but important adjustments not only in your food consumption, but in your understanding and attitude towards food and the way you view the role of physical activity in maintaining a healthy life. Each phase builds upon the previous phase like the levels of a pyramid that support the ones above it. The foundation and its integrity are what allow the peak to stand, so you must be careful in constructing the building blocks. A strong foundation will allow you to reach the top of your goals.

I have been shocked reading many diet books that say exercising is unnecessary or it's optional based on a dieter's preferences. One of the major reasons why so many people are overweight and obese and dying from preventable medical conditions such as heart disease is because we have become too sedentary! There are numerous studies from the best researchers in the world that show how important being physically active is not just for losing weight, but for becoming healthier and protecting things like our blood vessels, lungs and heart.

Studies also show that those who incorporate a regular exercise programme in their schedule will not only lose more weight faster, but will keep it off for longer periods of time. The problem that most people have is that they associate exercising with going to the gym and killing themselves for two hours, then dragging themselves home exhausted. That's *not* the exercise I'm talking about. Let's be realistic. It's not like you're training to become an Olympic gold medalist, right? What you need is a regular programme of physical activity that will keep your heart rate up and your lungs working. This will also help to tone your muscles and keep your joints active to help prevent certain illnesses like the dreaded arthritis. For each phase I give you very simple exercise suggestions to help you on your journey of becoming healthier and slimmer. Choose those exercises that you like and try to find a partner who is willing to do them with you. Studies have also shown that those who are most successful at losing weight have some type of support system in place – and a weight-loss partner makes exercise more fun!

The **FAT SMASH DIET** is about smashing the bad habits and demons of the past and constructing a new and improved you, now ready to take on fresh challenges and passions while fully enjoying the gift of life. Let's be perfectly clear. Diets are not magic. They are only blueprints. If you carefully follow the blueprint, then what you build can be magnificent. The **FAT SMASH DIET** is a blueprint that will help people trying to lose just 5 kilos (11 lb) as well as people trying to lose 100 kilos (220 lb). I'm extremely proud of this programme because it teaches the correct principles of healthy eating while at the same time allowing you to have a slice of cake or a couple of scoops of ice cream every now and again. Almost everything in life is about finding a balance and doing things in moderation. These are the underlying principles of The **FAT SMASH DIET**. You are now a SMASHER, so go SMASH IT!

Chapter 2
Phase I: **DETOX** (*9 days*)

This phase is ground zero, the beginning of the journey. The name 'detox' pretty much says it all. For the next nine days, you will eat mostly fruits and veggies and clean your body and mind of impurities naturally without fasting or putting any toxins into your system. This is about purifying your body and blood and feeding them the nutrients, vitamins and minerals that they so badly need. It's also about opening your mind and freeing it from the imprisonment of an unhealthy lifestyle. This is the first step towards a new you, so it's critical that you follow the principles of this phase and don't stray from the course.

Start by weighing yourself in the nude or a swim suit the morning you start this phase, then don't weigh yourself again until the morning of day 10. Have someone photograph you in a bathing costume. Take three shots with your hands hanging freely by your sides – a frontal shot, one from the side and the third from behind. Don't suck in your stomach; just stand naturally.

You need to record your healthy weight range, something that's indicated by your Body Mass Index (BMI). (You can find out how to do this in the appendix.) This is the measurement doctors now use to determine what you should weigh for your particular height.

Surround yourself with positive energy and people who are supportive of your new journey. Reduce stressful occurrences in your life: stress only distracts you from your important mission and induces poor decisions. Try not to think about food and weight constantly! Take up a hobby and enjoy life. Most important, get plenty of exercise. Medical studies prove that people who not only eat right but also exercise regularly (see page 24) not only lose weight faster but are most likely to keep it off permanently. If your mind isn't in the right place, then you won't be able to lose weight. Dieting is 50 per cent mental. Don't forget that!

And remember, cheating is a decision. If you do cheat, you are only cheating yourself. Now let's start SMASHING!

NUMBER OF MEALS PER DAY: (*4 or 5*)

These meals are designed in moderately sized portions. Don't stuff your plate as if you won't ever get to eat again. Now that you're eating more meals, you'll have less down time between meals, and you'll experience fewer hunger pangs. Because you'll be eating every 3–4 hours, you don't need to eat so much at each meal. It's important that you understand this. Even if you're not hungry, it's **critical** that you don't skip meals. Just eat a lighter meal. Your body needs to get into a comfortable not routine where it expects to be properly nourished at consistent time intervals.

WHAT TO EAT AND HOW MUCH:

During this detox phase you wil eat mostly fruits and veggies. You are allowed some other foods, as listed on page 21, but please note that the amounts given for these foods are the MAXIMUM alllowed! I strongly recommend that you not eat the maximum, and you need not eat them all. As for the fruits and veggies, simply eat the amount that fills you up, not so much that you feel stuffed. Remember, you're eating multiple small meals/snacks throughout the day, so there's no need to overeat.

MYTH:

If I skip meals or only eat once a day, I will lose weight because I'm eating fewer calories.

TRUTH:

The act of eating actually increases your metabolism, which helps you burn off the calories. When you don't eat, your body goes into 'starvation mode', which means your metabolism slows down and the calories that you do ingest are stored as fat. The body does this because fat is a great reserve of potential energy, to be used in the future when needed. When you skip meals and 'starve' yourself, the body doesn't know when it might see more food energy again, so it conserves and holds on to whatever it does see, storing it in the form of fat.

FOOD PREPARATION:

Foods are ONLY to be eaten raw, grilled, pan-grillled or steamed. You're allowed three tablespoons of low-fat dressing on your salads. If you're pan-grilling the veggies, use a minimal amount of olive oil (one to two teaspoons).

SAMPLE SCHEDULE:

Note: This is just a sample. You have to work out a schedule that fits your lifestyle, but keep in mind the spacing of the meals and the need to have at least four meals per day. For late-night snacks, try sliced fruit or raw/steamed veggies like celery, carrots, cucumbers, broccoli or asparagus.

8 am	Meal #1
11 am	Meal #2 *(heavy snack)*
2 pm	Meal #3
5 pm	Meal #4 *(light snack)*
7 pm	Meal #5
9 pm	Light Snack

DR. IAN'S TIP #1: Try frozen seedless grapes.
Put the grapes in the freezer, then grab them as you like.
They're delicious and low in calories!

DR. IAN'S TIP #2: Never eat within an hour and a half of going to bed. Try going for at least a 20- or 25-minute walk after dinner or participate in some other type of physical activity. This will help rev up your metabolism and burn off those calories before going to bed. It also releases endorphins, special chemicals in the body that make you feel good!

DR. IAN'S TIP #3: Eat foods high in fibre. Studies have shown that fibre helps to make you feel full longer, delays hunger pangs, reduces cholesterol levels, reduces constipation, reduces the risk of heart disease, and potentially helps prevent some intestinal cancers. Dietary sources of fibre include whole grains, fruits, vegetables, nuts and seeds.

FOOD/DRINKS ALLOWED: *(Phase I)*

- All fruits in any quantity
- All vegetables in any quantity, *except*:
  NO white potatoes
  NO avocados
- Good sources of protein:
  chickpeas
  beans
  tofu
  lentils
- Brown rice – 320 g (11 oz) of cooked rice per day
- 475 ml (17 fl oz) of semi-skimmed, skimmed or soya milk per day
- As much water as you like!
- Porridge – 160 g (5½ oz) per day
- All herbs and spices
- 90 g (3 oz) low-fat yoghurt (2 times per day)
- 4 egg whites per day
- 2 cups of herbal tea per day

FOOD/DRINKS NOT ALLOWED:

(Phase I)

- White rice
- Meat
- Fish
- Cheese
- Bread – all types
- Raisins
- Nuts
- Dried or preserved fruits
- Sweets/popcorn/crisps
- Ice cream
- Alcohol
- Juice
- Fizzy drinks – regular *or* diet
- Coffee and all coffee drinks
- Sports drinks
- Milkshakes
- Whole eggs or yolks
- Fried food
- Fast food

PHYSICAL ACTIVITY
At least 30 minutes of cardiovascular activity five days a week.

SAMPLE ACTIVITIES: NUMBER OF CALORIES
(*Burned Per Hour*)

Pilates (light) 200

Pilates (moderate) 300

Elliptical machine (moderate) 300

Tennis (singles) 350

Pilates (intense).................................400

Kickboxing 400–600

Dancing (aerobic) 420

Bicycle riding (moderate) 450

Power walking (3 mph) 450

Aerobics 450

Jogging (5 mph) 500

Swimming (active) 500

Hiking 500

Rowing (moderate effort) 550

Power Walking (intense effort).......................... 600

Basketball 700

Rowing (intense effort) 700

Running (11 to 30 min./mile) 700

Skipping rope (moderate – 70 jumps / min) 700

Elliptical machine (intense) 700

Skipping rope (intense – 125 jumps / min) 850

Running (10-min. mile) 850

Stair climbing (stadiums) 900

STRUCTURE: AT LEAST 30 minutes 5 days a week.
You can choose any five days you like. They don't have

to be consecutive and can include all, part, or none of the weekend. It's also fine to do more days if you like. Anything over five is a bonus! Keep a simple journal of the type of physical activity you engaged in, the time of day you did it and the amount of time you spent doing it.

SAMPLE SCHEDULE:

MON.	30 minutes – power walking (300 cal.)
TUES.	OFF DAY
WED.	30 minutes – elliptical (350 cal.)
THURS.	30 minutes – aerobics (225 cal.)
FRI.	OFF DAY
SAT.	30 minutes – stair climbing (450 cal.)
SUN.	30 minutes – cycling (225 cal.)

DR IAN'S TIP #4: Try to get your workout done early in the morning. It's a great start to the day and it takes the pressure off later, when you might be tired from a full day of work or busy with other plans. Also, if you work out early in the morning, you can always do some type of physical activity at night for a bonus!

DR. IAN'S TIP #5: While it's faster and more organised to meet your physical activity component by working out in a gym, you don't have to belong to a gym to make this programme work. Not everyone likes gyms and they can be costly. Try stair climbs or mini-stadiums. Go up and down a flight of stairs of at least 10 steps. Up and back down is considered 1 trip. Try to do at least 10 trips within 30 minutes with 30- to 45-second rest periods between each trip. If you don't want to make noise in the house, go to a local secondary athletic field.

DR. IAN'S TIP #6: CARDIO FAT BURNING

Work out with your heart rate in the fat-burning zone: 50–70% of maximum heart rate. Subtract your age from 220 to find your maximum heart rate. Then multiply that number by 0.5 – this will give you the minimum heart rate you should maintain while performing your physical activity. Then take your maximum heart rate and multiply it by 0.7 – this is the upper range for maximal fat burning.

EXAMPLE: (*40-year-old person*)

220 − 40 = 180 (maximum heart rate)

180 x 0.5 = 90 (lower limit of minimal fat-burning range)

180 x 0.7 = 126 (upper limit of maximal fat-burning range)

Range during exercise for maximal fat burning: 90–126 beats per minute

NOTE: THOSE WHO ARE BETTER CONDITIONED SHOULD WORK WITHIN THE RANGE OF 60–75% OF THEIR MAXIMUM HEART RATE.

Chapter 3
Phase II: FOUNDATION
(*3 weeks*)

CONGRATULATIONS! You have gone through the most difficult part of the programme: detoxification. Now that your body has detoxed and you have reintroduced the nourishing powers of fruits and vegetables to your diet, it's time to start laying the foundation to a healthier way of eating and a healthier you.

The purpose of this phase is to reintroduce many foods you missed during detox, those very foods your body was craving to eat. At this point it's important to remember that this is about SMASHING those bad habits of the past and building good habits for the future. It's important to stick to the guidelines of the programme with an understanding that you and your eating programme are a work in progress. Now is not the time to undo all of the progress you've made in Phase I, so some of the basic rules still apply: (1) do not overeat at any given sitting, but maintain the schedule of four or five smaller meals per day; (2) continue to eat as many fruits and vegetables as possible even though you are adding other foods to your diet; (3) DON'T skip meals and stick as closely as possible to the eating schedule that you've set up in Phase I, since this is what your body is now accustomed to following; (4) you MUST continue the physical activity portion of the programme as this will be the best way that you continue to burn off those calories and SMASH the fat; (5) continue to stay away from fried foods and fat-laden dressings that only add unnecessary calories and distribute bad fats in your blood.

Remember, we are building that pyramid and in order for the peak to tower beautifully in the sky, the blocks upon which it rests must remain strong and dependable. The blocks you put down in this phase are the most important since they are your FOUNDATION. Go SMASH it!

NUMBER OF MEALS PER DAY: (*4 or 5*)

It's EXTREMELY important that you eat at least four meals a day, because we are now adding more fun foods back in the diet and these fun foods pack a lot more calories than the fruits and vegetables of Phase I. Eating multiple meals will reduce the time you're waiting between meals and will help you to continue to cut down on the hunger pangs and cravings. Remember, it's all about smashing bad habits and building new ones. Setting a regular eating schedule is an important habit to develop! Maintain the smaller portions!

WHAT TO EAT AND HOW MUCH:

As in the previous phase, there's no limit to the amount of fruits and veggies you can eat at each meal, with the exception of avocados and potatoes. You are also allowed to have ONE serving of any of the lean meats listed on page 33 and ONE serving of the seafood. For example, you can have chicken breast (without the skin and the right size) for lunch and have a piece of salmon for a dinner meal. If you're allergic to seafood, then you should have two servings of meat that day – let's say chicken and turkey or whatever combination you prefer. If you don't want to eat meat, you can have two servings of the seafood. Remember that the amounts given are MAXIMUMS and that you're not expected to eat everything on the list every day!

This is not a diet where you have to sit down with a calculator and figure out how many calories you're consuming. Let hunger be your guide. Eat the fruits and veggies until the hunger is gone, but DON'T eat so much that you get up from the table feeling stuffed. This is essential. You will be re-energising yourself in no more than a few hours, so don't overdo it in one sitting.

Remember too, that more calories are coming back into your diet. You MUST do your exercise as prescribed in the book. If you don't exercise and you add all of those calories back, then you won't lose weight or – even worse – you might gain weight. So follow the diet and exercise programme strictly to continue getting results!

FOOD/DRINKS ALLOWED: *(Phase II)*

Vegetables and grains:

- Pak choi
- Broccoli
- Spring greens
- Dark green leafy lettuce
- Kale
- Mesclun
- Cos lettuce
- Spinach
- Watercress
- Acorn squash
- Butternut squash
- Carrots
- Pumpkin
- Sweet potatoes
- Black beans
- Black-eyed beans
- Chickpeas
- Kidney beans
- Lentils
- Sweetcorn
- Green peas

- Broad beans
- Artichokes
- Asparagus
- Bean sprouts
- Beetroot
- Brussels sprouts
- Cabbage
- Cauliflower
- Celery
- Cucumbers
- Aubergines
- Green beans
- Green/red peppers
- Mushrooms
- Okra
- Onions
- Parsnips
- Tomatoes
- Brown rice – 240 g (8½ oz) of cooked rice *every other day (if desired)*
- Avocado – ½ per day maximum

NOTE: These are total servings allowed per day; eat your servings during any meal you choose.

MEATS *90–115 g* *(3–4 oz).* (size of a deck of playing cards)	Chicken: baked without the skin (NO FRIED!) Turkey: baked without the skin Minced beef: EXTRA lean or minced sirloin, grilled Sirloin steak, grilled Lamb, grilled
SEAFOOD	Halibut, Tuna, Salmon, Sole, Halibut, etc.: 90 g (3 oz). (NO FRIED!) Prawns: 4 large Mussels: 85 g (3 oz). Oysters: 6–12 Clams: 3
EGGS	4 egg whites *plus* 1 whole egg—scrambled, boiled, or poached
MILK & CHEESE	570 ml (1 pt) of semi-skimmed, skimmed or soya milk Cheese: 30 g (1 oz) 180 g (6½ oz) low-fat yoghurt (2 times per day)

NEW

≫≫

CEREALS

cold
unsweetened
30g (1 oz) per day
hot
15g (½ oz) per day

Corn flakes
Cheerios
Porridge
Total
Bran flakes
Life
Rice Krispies
Puffed rice
Puffed wheat
Shredded wheat
Wheaties
Special K
Chex

SWEETENERS

4 tsp of granulated sugar
(or sugar substitute)

SPICES & HERBS

as you like!

Salt (2 tsp)
Pepper (as you like)

≫

➤➤

FLAVOURINGS	2 tbsp of fat-free dressing
	1 tbsp of extra virgin olive oil
	1 tbsp of fat-free mayo
	10 g (⅓ oz) of butter

DRINKS	1 285-ml (10 fl oz) cup of coffee
	3 cups of tea
	1.1 litres (2 pints) of soda water
	2 cans of diet fizzy drink
	230 ml (8 fl oz) of freshly squeezed fruit juice (you can divide this up into ½ cup servings)
	Iced tea – sweetened only with 2 packets of sugar substitute, such as Splenda
	Lemonade – made with real lemons and 2 packets of sugar substitute or 2 tsp of granulated sugar
	Tonic water, unlimited
	Unlimited tap or bottled water!

FOOD/DRINKS NOT ALLOWED:
(Phase II)

- White rice
- White potatoes
- Bread/Muffins
- White pasta or whole wheat pasta
- White flour
- Pastries/doughnuts/Danish pastry
- Cakes
- Biscuits
- Brownies
- Sweets
- Ice cream
- Potato crisps/tortilla chips/popcorn
- Chocolate
- Bacon
- Sausage
- Alcohol
- Fried food
- Fast food

>>

- Regular fizzy drinks
- Sweetened juices from a bottle or can
- Milkshakes
- Caffe latte or cappuccino

TIPS:

- Don't eat the same fish or meat twice in the same day

- Try to separate the meats by at least a meal

- Try to leave some of the food on your plate when you get up from the table

- Try to do some physical activity after eating dinner (at least 20 minutes)

- Snack only on fruits and veggies after dinner

- Remember portion size: less is more!

PHYSICAL ACTIVITY:

Same programme as Phase I, except it's time to KICK IT
UP because you're now eating a lot more calories, so you
must increase everything by 10–15 per cent.

For example: If you had walked for 30 minutes a
day, now walk for 35.

If you walked a mile a day, now walk 1.1–1.2 miles.

Remember, do the cardio exercises in your heart
range, which was explained in Phase I (page 27).

The more you do, the better!

No lifting free weights! (This will come in
Phase III or IV.)

SAMPLE SCHEDULE:

MON.	35 minutes – elliptical (408 cal.)
TUES.	35 minutes – swimming (291 cal.)
WED.	OFF DAY
THURS.	35 minutes – power walking (intense) (350 cal.)
FRI.	OFF DAY
SAT.	35 minutes – aerobics (263 cal.)
SUN.	35 minutes – skipping rope (408 cal.)

Chapter 4
Phase III: CONSTRUCTION
(*4 weeks*)

Over the last four weeks, you laid down a solid foundation for a healthier lifestyle that we will now continue to build on. Phase III will add more variety to your diet, constructing an eating plan that will allow you to enjoy many of the foods you've enjoyed in the past. The difference, however, is that with your greater understanding of portion control and the importance of more fruits and vegetables in your diet, you can now enjoy some of those sweets you've missed in the past, but instead of eating five biscuits, you'll be content with two. The first two phases instilled some important concepts that will guide your eating behaviours forever. Don't turn your back on all that you have learned and take up the old bad habits. Doing this will reverse the progress you've worked so hard to make.

Remember that you are now eating AT LEAST four times a day, which means you don't have to fill your plate to the rim, go back for seconds, or eat super-sized meals. Your body is now accustomed to consistency: the regular schedule of your eating times and the volume of food that you're consuming at one sitting. Do the best that you can not to disrupt this schedule, but if for some reason you can't maintain it, go back to it as soon as possible. A short interruption will not throw you too far off course. No dieter is perfect and at some point it is very likely that you might slip. This is not uncommon. It happens to almost everyone. If you slip, don't get anxious. The **FAT SMASH DIET** is designed to forgive, not punish. Simply go back on Phase I until you've lost any weight you have gained back. Once you've lost that weight, go an extra day on Phase I, then directly back to Phase III.

NUMBER OF MEALS PER DAY: (*4 or 5*)

QUANTITY OF FRUITS AND VEGGIES:

Let hunger be your guide. Eat enough that you're satisfied, not so much that you're stuffed. Remember, these foods are most nutritious when they're eaten raw, steamed, grilled, or baked. Frying is not permitted since this adds extra calories and destroys the nutrients contained in the food.

> **DR. IAN'S TIP :** Try one day of Phase I during each week of Phase III. This will cut the calories down for a few days and shake your body from its comfortable routine, which can kick-start more weight loss.

FOOD/DRINKS ALLOWED: *(Phase III)*

Vegetables and grains:

- Pak choi
- Broccoli
- Spring greens
- Dark green leafy lettuce
- Kale
- Mesclun
- Romaine lettuce
- Spinach
- Watercress
- Acorn squash
- Butternut squash
- Carrots
- Pumpkin
- Sweet potatoes
- Black beans
- Black-eyed peas
- Chickpeas
- Kidney beans
- Lentils
- Sweetcorn

- Green peas
- Broad beans
- Artichokes
- Asparagus
- Bean sprouts
- Beetroot
- Brussels sprouts
- Cabbage
- Cauliflower
- Celery
- Cucumbers
- Aubergines
- Green beans
- Green/red peppers
- Mushrooms
- Okra
- Onions
- Parsnips
- Tomatoes
- Brown rice – 320 g (11 oz) of cooked rice every other day (if desired)
- Avocado – 1/2 per day maximum

CEREALS
cold
unsweetened
30g (1 oz) per day
hot
15g (½ oz) per day

Corn flakes
Cheerios
Porridge
Bran flakes
Rice Krispies
Puffed rice
Puffed wheat
Shredded wheat
Special K

SWEETENERS

4 tsp of granulated sugar
(or sugar substitute)

**SPICES
&
HERBS**
as you like!

Salt (2 tsp)
Pepper (as you like)

FLAVOURINGS	2 tbsp of fat-free dressing 1 tbsp of extra virgin olive oil 1 tbsp of fat-free mayo 10 g (⅓ oz) of butter
DRINKS	1 285-ml (10 fl oz) cup of coffee with milk 3 cups of tea 1.1 litre (2 pints) of soda water 2 cans of diet fizzy drinks Iced tea – sweetened only with 2 packets of sugar substitute, such as Splenda Lemonade – made with real lemons and 2 packets of sugar substitute or 2 tsp of granulated sugar Tonic water, unlimited Unlimited tap or bottled water!

NEW

- 430 ml (¾ pint) of freshly squeezed fruit juice
(you can divide this up throughout the day as you like)

NEW

NOTE: These are total servings allowed per day; eat your servings during any meal you choose; the meat serving is now larger.

MEATS *140 g (5 oz)* size of a deck and a half of playing cards	Chicken: baked without the skin (NO FRIED!) Turkey: baked without the skin Minced beef: EXTRA lean or minced sirloin Sirloin steak, grilled Lamb, grilled Low-fat sausage
SEAFOOD	Halibut, Tuna, Salmon, Snapper, Striped Bass, etc.: 85 g (3 oz) (NO FRIED!) Prawns: 4 large Mussels: 85 g (3 oz) Oysters: 6–12 Clams: 3
EGGS	4 egg whites *plus* 2 whole eggs – scrambled, boiled or poached
MILK & CHEESE	570 ml (1 pt) of semi-skimmed, skimmed or soya milk Cheese: 35 g (1¼ oz)

PASTA & BREAD	Whole wheat pasta: 80 g (2¾ oz) per day Wholemeal/wholegrain bread: 4 thin slices
DESSERTS the serving size for the biscuits (except for digestives) is approximately 3.5 cm (1½ in)	Note: *one dessert per day at any meal you choose.* 3 chocolate chip cookies 4 ginger biscuits 2 oatmeal raisin biscuits 2 Garibaldi biscuits 2 large digestive biscuits 1 scoop of low-fat ice cream

FOOD/DRINKS NOT ALLOWED:
(Phase III)

- White rice
- White potatoes
- White bread/English muffins
- White pasta
- White flour
- Pastries/doughnuts/Danish pastries
- Cakes
- Brownies
- Sweets
- Potato crisps/tortilla chips/popcorn
- Bacon
- Sausage
- Alcohol
- Regular fizzy drinks
- Milkshakes
- Cappuccinos
- Caffe latte

PHYSICAL ACTIVITY:

Same programme as Phase II, except it's time to kick it up again; you're now eating a lot more calories, so you must increase everything by 25 per cent.

For example: if you were walking for 35 minutes a day, now walk for 45.

If you walked 1.1 miles a day, now walk 1.4 miles a day.

Remember, do the cardio exercises in your heart range, which was explained in Phase I (page 27).

Light free weights are optional, but it's better to do them in the next phase.

> **DR. IAN'S TIP :** Try to burn off some extra calories by doing a 'two-a-day'. This is what many well-conditioned athletes do. Work out twice in one day: a morning exercise routine and another in the evening. This will really rev up your metabolism.

SAMPLE SCHEDULE:

MON.	OFF DAY
TUES.	45 minutes – aerobics (338 cal.)
WED.	45 minutes – elliptical (525 cal.)
THURS.	OFF DAY
FRI.	45 minutes – basketball, full court (525 cal.)
SAT.	45 minutes – swimming (375 cal.)
SUN.	45 minutes – stair climbing (675 cal.)

Chapter 5
Phase IV: THE TEMPLE
(*for life*)

The fact that you've made it to this phase means that you have achieved tremendous success. This is no small feat. Be proud of yourself! You have **detoxed** your body, laid a solid **foundation** for a healthier way of living, and **constructed** a routine of good habits that will guide you throughout your life. All of this is like building a sacred temple, something to admire, respect and honour. But like any beautiful structure, there's also maintenance involved to keep it clean and shiny. Every once in a while there will be the need for minor repairs, and that's expected. The key, however, is to avoid the need for major fixes. This is where you are on The **FAT SMASH DIET**. Now that you've built the temple of good eating behaviours and a physical activity programme, you can admire and appreciate it, but also be prepared for minor tweaks as you go along. Remember that life is constantly evolving.

This phase is fluid in nature, since you never know

where the repairs need to be done or when. Maybe you've started eating too many sweet foods or increased the portions beyond the appropriate sizes. Some people will start slacking off on the physical activity regimen and will notice the weight slowly starting to creep back on. Don't get upset or frustrated. These are not major problems and they can be addressed very easily. That's the beauty of The **FAT SMASH DIET**. The important part is to identify the exact location of the leak in the roof and quickly use the necessary material to fix it. If you notice that you've gained back 10–15 per cent of the weight that you had lost earlier, then simply leave the temple (Phase IV), go back to detox (Phase I) until you've lost that weight again, then return directly to Phase IV, being mindful of your portions and keeping up your physical activity.

In this last phase, there are some food and beverage additions for you that will complete your eating programme. Since they've been absent from your diet for the last eight weeks, you can better appreciate them, but it's important to follow the guidelines and not overindulge. Remember, at this stage of the diet, you have SMASHED the bad habits and developed good, healthy habits through hard work and determination. This healthier way of living can sustain you as a lean, fit, healthy person forever.

DR. IAN'S TIP : Buy an inexpensive pedometer to keep track of how many steps you take per day. Try 6,000 steps for good health and 10,000 steps for weight loss.

NEW

NOTE: The foods from all of the previous phases are allowed in this phase. Just add from the chart below. Enjoy, but remember *PORTION CONTROL!*

BREAKFAST	Bacon – 4 strips per week Sausage – 1 per week 6 10 cm (4 in) pancakes per week (whole wheat is better) 2 medium-sized croissants per week

LUNCH & DINNER	2 slices of cheese pizza with
	    any toppings – twice a week
	White rice – 2 servings a week
	    (but brown is still better)
	1 white jacket potato a week
	    (but sweet potato is still better)
	2 small servings of chips per week
	1 serving of ricotta cheese three
	    times per week
	Cheddar, Port Salut, or Red Leicester
	    cheese, 2 35g slices per day
	2 medium-sized crab cakes per week
	1 medium-sized lobster per week
	    (use butter sparingly!)
	4 medium slices of ham per week
	    (avoid the fat)

>>

❯❯

DRINKS	2 230-ml (8 oz) cups of fizzy drink per week (diet drinks are much better)
	2 pints of beer per week (preferably not at one sitting)
	3 glasses of wine per week (preferably not at one sitting)
	3 230 ml (8 oz) caffe lattes or cappuccinos per week (try using skimmed milk)
	1 340 ml (12 oz) milkshake per week

PHYSICAL ACTIVITY:

By this point you should be in a comfortable excercise routine. Exercise five times a week for one intense hour each time. It's very important to change your workout routine, since your body can quickly become accustomed to your exercise schedule and stop burning the calories.

Also, start lifting light free weights under supervision. This will help build up your lean muscle mass. You should lift weights at least twice a week, working on your different body parts. You can do this right at home with dumbbells. But you should make sure you have been trained on the proper lifting techniques before attempting them.

Continuing your physical activity plan is ESSENTIAL for you to develop the complete package. It will only boost the results you obtain on the diet!

Chapter 6
BUSTING THROUGH THE PLATEAU

Almost everyone over the course of a diet hits a plateau, a point where they can't seem to lose weight any more despite their previous success. This is what I call the critical point. It's critical, because unfortunately, most people get frustrated and disappointed and quit. DON'T QUIT! Plateaus are very natural and happen for a good reason. The body is an extremely clever machine, and while we think that we can fool it, we can only do so for short periods of time at most. The body becomes accustomed to your new way of eating and your exercise regimen and decides that it is not going to keep burning calories by shedding fat. Believe it or not, that's an important protective feature of how our bodies operate. Imagine if you were stuck on a cold mountain with no way of getting food or water for a prolonged period of time. The body works to conserve your fat – the source of energy – as long as possible so that you can last without food and water until a rescue team arrives. Well, it's that feature that kicks in when you've been doing so well losing weight.

But there is a way to bust through this 'standstill' point and it requires patience and determination. First, each time you exercise, increase it by 20 per cent and do this for nine days. For example, if you normally walk for 60 minutes during your exercise time, walk for 72 minutes instead. If you normally walk 2 miles at a time, walk 2.4 miles. At the same time, decrease the amount of calories you consume by eating smaller portions. This way, you're attacking the problem from both ends.

Another method is to change your diet altogether. Sometimes you have to 'shock' the system to get it going. So go back to an earlier phase like I or II or a combination of them and stay there for seven days. You can play with the combination as you like, but the idea is to do something different from what you've been doing. You should also change your exercise programme. Try to do a different exercise. If you spend most of your time walking, then try doing stairs or playing a sport. Don't decrease your time, just switch up the activity.

The bottom line is that in order to bust through the plateau, you must shake your body out of its comfort zone. Do this for 7–9 days and you will get through it. There's no universal solution that works for everyone, but I have found these strategies to be very effective for most dieters I've helped over the years.

SAMPLE SCHEDULE:

MON.	60 minutes – elliptical (700 cal.)
TUES.	60 minutes – swimming (500 cal.)
WED.	OFF DAY
THURS.	60 minutes – power walking (intense) (600 cal.)
FRI.	OFF DAY
SAT.	60 minutes – aerobics (450 cal.)
SUN.	60 minutes – skipping rope, 70 jumps /min (700 cal.)

Chapter 7
TASTY RECIPES

** Most recipes provided by Big City Chefs: **www.bigcitychefs.com***

NOTE: Look carefully at the serving sizes for the different recipes. In many cases it's four or more for that particular recipe, which means you are not to eat all of it. You are still ONLY to have one serving size per meal at most! Remember, this is about portion control. You are eating more meals per day, which means each meal MUST be smaller or you'll be packing in too many calories! Stow away the extra portions in individual containers for later in the week or stash them in the freezer for the next phase of the programme.

For those readers who may lack the time or ability to prepare the recipes in this book, or for those who may enjoy an additional selection of recipes consistent with Dr. Ian's nutritional guidelines, contact Big City Chefs at www.bigcitychefs.com. Big City Chefs staffs professionally trained personal chefs in major metropolitan regions across the United States, providing personalised menu planning and in-home preparation of one to two weeks of meals per visit.

PHASE I | Sample Recipes

GOOD BREAKFAST HABITS

_____

_____

_____

_____

_____

_____

_____

_____

_____

_____

BAD BREAKFAST HABITS

_____

_____

_____

_____

_____

_____

_____

_____

_____

_____

_____

Breakfast | (*Phase I*)

Recipes on the go!

- 80   g (2¾ oz) porridge
  115   g (4 oz) of raspberries
  115   ml (4 fl oz) semi-skimmed
      milk

- ½   cantaloupe melon
  180   g (6½ oz) low-fat yoghurt
  225   ml (8 fl oz) of fresh orange
      juice

- 4   egg whites, beaten
  ½   red grapefruit
  230   ml (8 fl oz) milk

Lunch | (*Phase I*)

(Green Bean Salad)

Serves : 4–6

450 g (1 lb) fresh green beans, trimmed
10 cherry tomatoes, halved
1 yellow pepper, seeded
     and cut into julienne strips
½ large green pepper (approx. 60 g [2 oz]), chopped
3 rounded tbsp chopped fresh parsley

For dressing :
1 tsp Dijon mustard
55 ml (2 fl oz) cup olive oil
55 ml (fl oz) cup fresh lemon juice
¼ tsp freshly ground pepper
1 pinch salt

INSTRUCTIONS

Wash beans thoroughly. Drop the green beans into a saucepan of boiling water. Cook until slightly crisp, about four minutes.

Drain off water and let beans cool. Add tomatoes, peppers, and parsley.

To make the dressing : Combine mustard, oil, and lemon juice in a small bowl. Stir well.

Then add pepper and salt and stir again.

Lightly pour the dressing over the salad, then toss. Transfer the salad to a serving bowl, cover, and refrigerate for at least an hour until well chilled.

Vigorous Vegetable Soup

Serves : 4

1	medium courgette, chopped
100	g (3½ oz) mushrooms, chopped
1	medium onion, chopped
7	large carrots, chopped
4	celery sticks, chopped
1	sprig rosemary
1	tsp dried thyme
1	bay leaf
¼	tsp crushed red pepper flakes
285	g (10 oz) package frozen green peas, thawed
400	ml (14 fl oz) cans low-fat, low-sodium beef broth (or vegetable broth)
700	ml (1¼ pt) water

INSTRUCTIONS

Place all the ingredients except the peas in a large pot with the water, broth, and spices.

Bring to a boil, then let simmer for 45 minutes or until carrots are tender. Add peas for last 5 minutes of cooking time.

Remove the bay leaf and rosemary sprig before serving.

Carrot Soup

Serves : 4

5   g (⅙ oz) butter
10   carrots, chopped
1   small onion, chopped
1.2   litres (2 pints) of vegetable
     stock or beef stock
3   tbsp curry powder
50   g (1¾ oz) brown rice (optional)
1   tbsp finely chopped ginger
2   cloves garlic, finely chopped
    Sprig of parsley
    Bay leaves
    Salt and pepper

INSTRUCTIONS

Melt butter in medium frying pan. Add carrots
and onion and sauté until soft, approximately
10–15 minutes.

Next add the remaining ingredients, bring to a
boil, and simmer for 30–40 minutes.

Remove parsley and bay leaves, then pour mix
into a blender in batches and puree.

Serve hot or cold.

Dinner | (*Phase I*)

Lentils with Grilled Mushrooms, Asparagus and Asparagus Broth

Serves : 4

200	g (7 oz) mushrooms
3	tbsp olive oil
500	g (1 lb 2 oz) cooked lentils
1	clove garlic, finely chopped
130	g (4½ oz) asparagus, steamed and chopped
2	tbsp fresh basil, cut into chiffonade (thin strips)
	Salt and pepper to taste

For asparagus broth :

2	tsp olive oil
30	g (1 oz) each carrot, onion and celery, chopped
2	cloves garlic, whole
2	tbsp white wine
70	g (2½ oz) asparagus ends, roughly chopped (*use leftover woody ends of stems that are not used above*)
700	ml (1¼ pint) vegetable broth
1	bay leaf
	Basil stems (*from basil above*)
	Salt and pepper to taste

INSTRUCTIONS

To make the asparagus broth : Heat olive oil over medium heat and sweat carrot, onion, celery and garlic cloves for approximately 2 minutes. Add white wine and cook for 1 minute. Add asparagus ends, broth, bay leaf and basil stems. Reduce heat and simmer for 20 minutes. Strain and set aside.

Toss mushrooms with 2 tablespoons of the olive oil and pan-grill them on medium heat for 2 minutes per side (you may alternatively oven-roast them on a baking sheet for 10 minutes at 200°C/400°F/Gas mark 6). Let mushrooms cool, then slice. Heat 1 tbsp olive oil in a sauté pan over high heat, add garlic and briefly sweat until aromas are released. Add lentils, mushrooms and asparagus and cook for 1 minute over high heat. Add asparagus broth and bring to a simmer. Heat through until all ingredients are hot. Remove from the heat, add the basil, season with salt and pepper and serve.

NUTRITIONAL INFORMATION:

Per Serving : 417 Calories; 14g Fat (29.2% calories from fat); 20g Protein; 56g Carbohydrate; 16g Dietary Fibre; 2mg Cholesterol; 1,235mg Sodium. Exchanges: 3 Grain (Starch); 1 Lean Meat; 1 Vegetable; 3 Fat.

(Sweetcorn Salad)

Serves : 4

3	ml portobello mushrooms, chopped
70	ml (2½ fl oz) balsamic vinegar
70	ml (2½ fl oz) olive oil
4	tsp water
	Pinch of brown or white sugar
230	g (8 oz) frozen sweetcorn, thawed and drained
200	g (7 oz) cherry tomatoes, halved
1	medium onion, chopped
115–230	g (4–8 oz) baby lettuce leaves
1	green pepper, chopped
6	rounded tbsp chopped fresh parsley
6	rounded tbsp chopped chives (optional)
	Salt and pepper to taste

INSTRUCTIONS

Marinate the mushrooms for 45 minutes in vinegar, olive oil, water and sugar.

While mushrooms marinate, mix sweetcorn, tomatoes, onion, lettuce, pepper, parsley, chives, salt and pepper in a large bowl.

Drizzle the marinated mushrooms over the salad or keep to the side and dip.

Pan-grilled Vegetable Platter

Serves : 4

2	yellow peppers
2	red peppers
3	courgettes, halved lengthwise
3	squash, halved lengthwise
18	asparagus spears, tough ends trimmed
4	tomatoes

For dressing (*makes about 230 ml [8 fl oz]*) :

170	ml (6 fl oz) olive oil
3	tbsp balsamic vinegar
2	cloves garlic, finely chopped
1	tsp fresh lemon juice
	Pinch dried basil
	Pinch dried oregano
	Salt and freshly ground pepper

INSTRUCTIONS

To make the dressing : Mix the ingredients together in a small bowl. Set aside.

Slice the vegetables and pan-grill them over medium heat using a small amout of low-fat oil. Cook peppers until slightly charred. Cook courgettes and squash about 4 minutes on each side. Cook asparagus for about 5 minutes total. Cook tomatoes for about 3 minutes on each side.

Drizzle vegetables lightly with dressing.

Chilled Asparagus with
Rosemary and Lemon Vinaigrette

Serves : 4–6

2	tsp fresh lemon juice
2	tbsp red wine vinegar
2	tbsp finely chopped fresh rosemary
2	cloves garlic
1	tsp low-fat mayonnaise
115	ml (4 fl oz) extra virgin olive oil
30	asparagus spears, peeled and tough ends trimmed
	Light sprinkle salt and pepper

INSTRUCTIONS

Combine lemon juice, vinegar, rosemary, garlic and mayonnaise in a small bowl. Whisk in the olive oil slowly to create a creamy sauce. Season with salt and pepper.

Bring a large saucepan of water to a boil and add asparagus. Boil until tender. Remove the asparagus, then shock it in ice water (4 litres [7 pints] of water and three trays of ice) for about 2 minutes to stop the asparagus from cooking.

Drain asparagus again and place on paper towels and pat dry. Then arrange the asparagus on a serving platter. Cover and refrigerate about 1 hour until completely chilled.

When it's time to serve, pour vinaigrette evenly over the asparagus.

(Tasty Tomatoes)

Serves : 4–6

4	medium tomatoes
2	tsp finely chopped chives
3	tbsp low-fat mayonnaise
1½	tsp Dijon mustard
	Light sprinkle salt and pepper
4	tbsp grated Parmesan cheese

INSTRUCTIONS

Preheat the oven to 190°C/375°F/Gas mark 5.

Cut tomatoes in half horizontally and place cut side up on a baking tray.

In a bowl, stir the topping : chives, mayonnaise, mustard, salt and pepper, and 2 tablespoons of the Parmesan cheese. Once the topping is nicely mixed, scoop out small amounts with a spoon and place on top of the tomatoes.

Take the rest of the cheese and sprinkle on top. Then bake for 10 minutes or until the tomatoes are hot. Once this is done, quickly put the tomatoes into the grill for a minute to get the topping really brown and hot.

Serve hot.

WHAT WAS EASY IN PHASE I

_____
_____
_____
_____
_____
_____
_____
_____
_____
_____
_____
_____
_____

WHAT WAS DIFFICULT IN PHASE I

_____
_____
_____
_____
_____
_____
_____
_____
_____
_____
_____
_____

PHASE II | Sample Recipes

NEW FOODS THAT YOU'VE COME TO LIKE

_____

_____

_____

_____

_____

_____

_____

_____

_____

_____

_____

_____

_____

_____

_____

_____

_____

_____

_____

_____

_____

_____

_____

_____

_____

Breakfast | (*Phase II*)

Recipes on the go!

- 70 g (2½ oz) bran cereal
  230 ml (8 fl oz) semi-skimmed milk
  1 medium banana
  230 ml (8 fl oz) orange juice

- 20 g (¾ oz) puffed wheat
  230 ml (8 fl oz) semi-skimmed milk
  ¼ cantaloupe melon

- 2 boiled eggs
  180 g (6½ oz) plain yoghurt
  230 ml (8 fl oz) semi-skimmed milk

Lunch | (*Phase II*)

Kidney Beans with Sautéed Prawns and Asparagus

Serves : 4

340	g (12 oz) raw prawns, peeled and deveined
1	tbsp olive oil
1	clove garlic, finely chopped
400	g (14 oz) kidney beans, cooked and drained, or use rinsed beans
2	tbsp white wine
500	ml (18 fl oz) cups vegetable stock
300	g (10½ oz) cups steamed and chopped asparagus
1	tbsp finely chopped fresh basil
1	tbsp finely chopped fresh thyme
	Salt and pepper to taste

For marinade :

2	tbsp fresh lemon juice
2	tsp finely chopped fresh thyme
4	tbsp basil, cut into chiffonade (thin strips)
1	tbsp extra virgin olive oil
	Salt and pepper to taste

INSTRUCTIONS

Combine marinade ingredients, add prawns, and let stand in refrigerator for 20 minutes. Drain marinade and discard.

In a sauté pan, heat 1 tbsp olive oil over high heat and cook prawns for 2 minutes per side.

Add garlic and briefly sweat until aromas are released.

Add kidney beans and white wine and cook for 1 minute over high heat.

Add the stock, bring to a simmer, and add the asparagus.

Heat through until all ingredients are hot and prawns are a white, opaque colour.

Remove from heat, add the fresh herbs, season to taste with salt and pepper, and serve.

NUTRITIONAL INFORMATION:

Per Serving : 429 Calories; 11g Fat (23.0% calories from fat); 33g Protein; 49g Carbohydrate; 12g Dietary Fibre; 131mg Cholesterol; 945mg Sodium. Exchanges: 3 Grain (Starch); 3 Lean Meat; ½ Vegetable; 0 Fruit; 2 Fat.

Greek Vegetable Stew with Chickpeas

Serves : 4

1	tbsp olive oil
240	g (8½ oz) chopped onion
2	large green peppers, chopped
200	g (7 oz) sliced mushrooms
230	g (8 oz) artichoke hearts, sliced (can use frozen or tinned if fresh are not available)
1	tsp cumin
1	pinch cinnamon
2	tbsp finely chopped garlic
1.4	litres (2½ pints) vegetable stock
700	g (1½ lb) plum tomatoes, chopped Salt and pepper to taste
320	g (11 oz) chickpeas, cooked, or use rinsed tinned beans
1	tbsp lemon juice
100	g (3½ oz) Kalamata olives, pitted and sliced
1	tbsp finely chopped fresh oregano
2	tbsp finely chopped mint
2	tbsp finely chopped dill
60	g (2 oz) crumbled feta cheese

INSTRUCTIONS

In a sauté pan, heat olive oil over high heat and add onion, green pepper, mushrooms, artichokes, cumin and cinnamon. Cook until golden brown, approximately 5 minutes, stirring occasionally.

Add garlic and stir. Cook for 20–30 seconds until the aromas are released.

Add stock and simmer for 15 minutes.

Add tomatoes and chickpeas and simmer for an additional 5 minutes.

Remove from heat. Add the lemon juice, olives and herbs and serve in bowls, garnished with crumbled feta.

NUTRITIONAL INFORMATION:

Per Serving : 652 Calories; 22g Fat (28.7% calories from fat); 26g Protein; 96g Carbohydrate; 17g Dietary Fibre; 20mg Cholesterol; 3,071mg Sodium. Exchanges: 4 Grain (Starch); 1 Lean Meat; 5½ Vegetable; 0 Fruit; 4 Fat.

Seafood Gumbo with Brown Rice

Serves : 4

80	ml (2¾ oz) olive oil
45	g (1½ oz) whole wheat flour
115	g (4 oz) diced onion
3	cloves garlic, finely chopped
120	g (4¼ oz) chopped celery
1	very large (approx 130 g [4½ oz] green pepper, chopped
450	g (1 lb) raw seafood, in any combination of fish or prawns
3	tbsp filé powder
1	tbsp cayenne pepper
1.4	litres (2½ pints) vegetable stock
100	g (3½ oz) okra
230	g (8 oz) chopped tomatoes
1	tbsp each fresh oregano, basil and thyme finely chopped
	Salt and pepper to taste
200	g (7 oz) brown rice
1	litre (1¾ pints) water
	Salt and pepper to taste

INSTRUCTIONS

First make the roux. In a large saucepan, heat olive oil over medium-low heat and add flour. Stir into a paste and cook for several minutes, stirring, until a rich nutty brown colour develops.

Add onion, garlic, celery and green pepper to roux and cook for approximately 2 minutes, stirring constantly. Roux will cling to vegetables.

Add seafood and cook for approximately 3 minutes. Add filé powder and cayenne pepper. Add chicken stock and bring mixture to a simmer for ten minutes, stirring constantly.

Add okra, tomatoes and herbs and cook for 5 minutes.

Season to taste with salt and pepper. Serve over brown rice.

To make brown rice, bring rice, 1 litre (1¾ pints) of water, and salt to a boil in an uncovered pot. Then reduce heat to low, cover and simmer for approximately 45 minutes.

My Mother's Yummy Teriyaki Green Beans

Serves : 4

450 g (1 lb) frozen green beans
2 tbsp olive oil
60 ml (2 fl oz) of Amoy reduced salt
     teriyaki grilling sauce
230 ml (8 fl oz) Kikkoman stir-fry sauce
3 tbsp of sweet and sour
     stir-fry sauce
2 splashes of Worcestershire sauce
2 splashes of soy sauce
2 splashes of Kikkoman
     teriyaki sauce

INSTRUCTIONS

Heat oil in a wok or frying pan until very hot.

Drop frozen beans into oil and turn immediately to coat beans with oil.

Add the remaining ingredients and stir until well coated.

Cook on low heat until tender, approximately 15 minutes.

Season to taste.

Chopped Vegetable Salad

Serves : 4–6

1   large cucumber, peeled and sliced
150   g (5 oz) cherry tomatoes, sliced in half
2   spring onions, finely chopped
    (optional)
1   green pepper, chopped
230   g (8 oz) chopped fresh French beans
70   g (2½ oz) cooked sweetcorn
2   carrots, chopped or thinly sliced
2   tsp finely chopped chives

For dressing :
80   ml (2¾ fl oz) extra virgin olive oil
80   ml (2¾ fl oz) balsamic vinegar
½   tsp finely chopped garlic
    Salt and pepper to taste

INSTRUCTIONS

Mix the cucumbers, tomatoes, spring onions, pepper, beans, sweetcorn, carrots and chives in a large bowl.

To make the dressing : In smaller bowl, mix oil, vinegar, garlic, salt and pepper. Stir well.

Pour dressing over vegetables. Chill for fifteen minutes in refrigerator, then serve.

Dinner | (*Phase II*)

Chickpeas with Chicken, Broccoli and Tomato Broth

Serves : 4–6

2   tbsp fresh lemon juice

2   tsp finely chopped fresh oregano

4   tbsp fresh basil, cut into chiffonade (thin strips)

1   tbsp extra virgin olive oil

    Salt and pepper to taste

2   boneless, skinless chicken breasts, cut into julienne strips

1   tbsp olive oil

1   clove garlic, finely chopped

500   g (1 lb 2 oz) cooked chickpeas or use, rinsed tinned beans

460   g (1 lb) broccoli florets, steamed and chopped

For tomato broth :

1   tbsp olive oil

30   g (1 oz) each chopped carrot, onion and celery

2   cloves garlic

1   tbsp white wine

3   plum tomatoes, chopped

700   ml (1¼ pints) chicken broth

1   bay leaf

    Basil stems (*from basil above*)

    Salt and pepper to taste

INSTRUCTIONS

To make the tomato broth : Heat olive oil over medium heat and sweat carrots, onion, celery and garlic cloves for approximately 2 minutes. Add white wine and cook for 1 minute. Add tomatoes, broth, bay leaf and basil stems. Reduce heat and simmer for 20 minutes. Strain, season with salt and pepper and set aside.

Combine lemon juice, 1 tsp of the oregano, 2 tsp of the basil, and the extra virgin olive oil. Add to chicken and let stand in refrigerator for 20 minutes. Drain.

To make the chicken : Heat 1 tbsp olive oil in a sauté pan over high heat and cook chicken until fully cooked (test one piece by cutting into it). Add garlic and briefly sweat until aromas are released.

Add chickpeas and cook for 1 minute over high heat. Add tomato broth, bring to a simmer, and add broccoli. Heat through until all ingredients are hot.

Remove from the heat, add remaining oregano and basil, season to taste with salt and pepper, and serve.

NUTRITIONAL INFORMATION:

Per Serving : 486 Calories; 15g Fat (28.9% calories from fat); 41g Protein; 45g Carbohydrate; 7g Dietary Fibre; 68mg Cholesterol; 1,724mg Sodium. Exchanges: 2 Grain (starch); 4½ Lean Meat; ½ Vegetables; 0 Fruit; 2 1/2 Fat.

Roasted Sea Bass

Serves : 4

30 g (1 oz) fresh breadcrumbs
   (optional for Phase II)
1 clove garlic, finely chopped
3 tbsp chopped fresh parsley
2 tbsp finely chopped fresh basil
2 tbsp drained capers (optional)
1 tsp Dijon mustard
1 tbsp fresh lemon juice
   Salt and freshly ground pepper to taste
3 tbsp extra virgin olive oil
115 g (4 oz) sea bass fillets without the
   skin

INSTRUCTIONS

Preheat the oven to 180° C/350°F/Gas mark 7.

Mix breadcrumbs, garlic, parsley, basil, capers, mustard, lemon juice, salt and pepper in a small bowl.

In a frying pan over high heat, sauté the sea bass in the oil for about 1–2 minutes on each side.

Apply the breadcrumb mix to each fillet and make sure it adheres. Place the fillets on a rack set in a roasting pan.

Cook for about 10 minutes, to your preference.

WHAT WAS EASY IN PHASE II

_____

_____

_____

_____

_____

_____

_____

_____

_____

_____

_____

WHAT WAS DIFFICULT IN PHASE II

_____

_____

_____

_____

_____

_____

_____

_____

_____

_____

_____

_____

PHASE III | Sample Recipes

ALL GOOD HABITS LEARNED IN PHASES I & II

Breakfast | (*Phase III*)

Recipes on the go!

- 1 English muffin, toasted
  2 tsp peanut butter
  180 g (6 ½ oz) plain low-fat
       yoghurt
  80 g (2¾ oz) blackberries

- ½ bagel, toasted
  4 egg whites, beaten
  230 ml (8 fl oz) fresh orange juice

- 2 eggs, scrambled
  1 English muffin
  5 g (⅙ oz) butter
  230 ml (8 fl oz) fresh orange juice

Country Breakfast Cake
with Porridge and Side Dish of Fruit

Serves : 4

230   g (8 oz) minced turkey
2   eggs
2   tbsp chopped red pepper
2   tbsp chopped yellow onion
1   tsp minced fresh thyme
     Salt and pepper to taste
1   tbsp olive oil
55   g (2 oz) dry instant oats
230   ml (8 fl oz) skimmed milk
160   g (5½ oz) strawberries, sliced

INSTRUCTIONS

Combine minced turkey, eggs, pepper, onion, thyme, salt and pepper and form into 4 cakes.

Heat the olive oil in a frying pan and fry cakes until cooked through and golden brown on both sides, approximately 3 minutes on each side, depending on the thickness of the cakes.

Cook oats in milk according to packet instructions.

Serve cake accompanied by sliced strawberries and porridge.

NUTRITIONAL INFORMATION:

Per Serving : 224 Calories; 11g Fat (46.1% calories from fat); 17g Protein; 13g Carbohydrate; 2g Dietary Fibre; 152mg Cholesterol; 223mg Sodium. Exchanges: ½ Grain (Starch); 2 Lean Meat; 0 Vegetable; 0 Fruit; 0 Skimmed Milk; 1 Fat.

Tropical Fruit Salad with Prosciutto

Serves : 4

2   slices prosciutto
45 g (1½ oz) pineapple, peeled,
    cored and chopped
45 g (1½ oz) mango, pitted,
    peeled and chopped
45 g (1½ oz) papaya, pitted,
    peeled and chopped
45 g (1½ oz) banana, sliced
55 g (2 oz) strawberries, sliced
55 g (2 oz) kiwi fruit, peeled
    and sliced
    Mint leaves for garnish

INSTRUCTIONS

Preheat oven to 200°C/400°F/Gas mark 6

To make the fruit salad · Combine fruit and toss.

Cut the prossiutto slices in half and serve with
fruit salad, garnished with mint leaf.

NUTRITIONAL INFORMATION:

Per Serving : 185 Calories; 11g Fat (52.8% calories from fat); 9g Protein;
14g Carbohydrate; 2g Dietary Fibre; 45mg Cholesterol; 382mg Sodium.
Exchanges: 1 Lean Meat; 1 Fruit; 1½ Fat.

Poached Eggs and Spinach on English Muffin with Tomato-Mint Coulis

Serves : 4

1	tsp olive oil
½	clove garlic, finely chopped
1	tbsp chopped onion
2	plum tomatoes, roughly chopped
1	tsp red wine vinegar
	Salt and pepper
1	tbsp finely chopped mint
2	tsp white vinegar
4	wholemeal English muffins, split
8	large eggs
330	g (12 oz) spinach, steamed

INSTRUCTIONS

To make the coulis : In a saucepan, heat olive oil over medium heat and sweat garlic and onion until translucent. Add tomatoes and cook for 10 minutes. Add vinegar and simmer for an additional 2 minutes. Season to taste with salt and pepper, remove from heat, and purée in a food processor until smooth. Add fresh mint.

In a stockpot or large saucepan, bring 4 litres (7 pints) of water and the white vinegar to a low simmer.

Toast the English muffins.

Carefully crack the eggs directly into the water and vinegar mixture, and let cook for 4 minutes. Remove them with a slotted spoon.

Spoon warm spinach over muffins, top with eggs and spoon coulis over eggs.

NUTRITIONAL INFORMATION:

Per Serving : 311 Calories; 13g Fat (35.9% calories from fat); 19g Protein; 31g Carbohydrate; 5g Dietary Fibre; 424mg Cholesterol; 578mg Sodium. Exchanges: 1 1/2 Grain (Starch); 1½ Lean Meat; ½ Vegetable; 1 Fat; 0 Other Carbohydrates.

Mushroom, Pepper and Cheddar Frittata with Macerated Fresh Berries

Serves : 4

For berries :

230	g (8 oz) mixed blueberries, strawberries, raspberries and blackberries
1	tbsp granulated sugar substitute (Splenda recommended)
1	tbsp lemon juice

For frittata :

1	red pepper, chopped
100	g (3½ oz) sliced mushrooms
1	tsp olive oil
4	large eggs
14	egg whites
	Salt and pepper to taste
4	thin slices Cheddar cheese
1	tbsp grated Parmesan cheese

INSTRUCTIONS

Preheat the oven to 250°C/500°F/Gas mark 10.

To macerate the berries : Toss them with the sugar substitute and lemon juice. Let stand while you make the frittata.

To make the frittata : In a small sauté pan, sauté red pepper and mushrooms in ½ teaspoon of the olive oil over high heat for about 2 minutes or until softened. Whisk together whole eggs and egg whites, and season to taste with salt and pepper.

In a separate oven-proof sauté pan, heat remaining olive oil over high heat and add eggs, stirring every minute for a total of approximately 5 minutes, or until eggs are set.

Layer the red pepper and mushrooms, Cheddar and Parmesan on top of the frittata and place the pan in the oven (or under the grill) for 2 minutes.

Cut into wedges and serve hot with the berries.

NUTRITIONAL INFORMATION:

Per Serving : 250 Calories; 11g Fat (38.6% calories from fat); 24g Protein; 14g Carbohydrate; 4g Dietary Fibre; 223mg Cholesterol; 418mg Sodium. Exchanges: 3 Lean Meat; ½ Vegetable; ½ Fruit; 1 Fat; 0 Other Carbohydrates.

Lunch | (*Phase III*)

(Hearty Black Bean Soup)

Serves : 8

455	g (1 lb) black beans, soaked in water overnight or for at least 6 hours
2	medium onions, chopped
2	small carrots, chopped
1	celery stick, chopped
4	tsp extra virgin olive oil
4	cloves garlic, finely chopped
½	tsp dried oregano
½	tsp cumin
1	tsp soy sauce
1	tbsp fresh lemon juice

INSTRUCTIONS

Drain the beans. Put them on a large pot and add water to cover. Simmer beans until they are soft, about 1½ hours.

Sauté onion, celery and carrot in olive oil. Add garlic, oregano, cumin and soy sauce. Cook, stirring, for 5 minutes.

Add the vegetables to the beans.

Cook for another 30 minutes. Add more water if necessary.

Just before serving, add the lemon juice.

Chicken and Summer Vegetable Broth

Serves : 4

70	g (2½ oz) lentils
1	bay leaf
2.2	litres (3¾ pints) chicken stock
½	aubergine, chopped
1	courgette, chopped
1	yellow squash, chopped
1	red pepper, chopped
115	g (4 oz) plum tomatoes, chopped
115	g (4 oz) French beans
	Salt and pepper to taste
1	tbsp finely chopped fresh basil
1	tsp finely chopped fresh parsley
1	tsp finely chopped fresh thyme

INSTRUCTIONS

Simmer lentils and bay leaf in chicken stock for 40 minutes.

Add the aubergine, courgette, yellow squash, pepper, tomatoes, beans, salt and pepper and simmer for 15 minutes.

Add fresh herbs and serve immediately.

NUTRITIONAL INFORMATION:

Per Serving : 171 Calories; 1g Fat (5.9% calories from fat); 11g Protein; 26g Carbohydrate; 11g Dietary Fibre; 0mg Cholesterol; 4304mg Sodium. Exchanges: 1 Grain(Starch); ½ Lean Meat; 2 Vegetable.

Dinner | (*Phase III*)

Black Beans with Herb-Marinated Chicken and Marinated Roasted Peppers

Serves : 4

2	boneless, skinless chicken breasts, cut into julienne strips
2	tbsp olive oil
1	tbsp finely chopped fresh oregano
2	tbsp finely chopped coriander
3	tbsp lemon juice
1	tsp chilli powder
1	tsp cumin
400	g (14 oz) cooked black beans, or use rinsed tinned beans
2	red peppers, roasted, peeled, seeded and sliced
1	green pepper, roasted, peeled, seeded and sliced
1	yellow pepper, roasted, peeled, seeded and sliced
30	g (1 oz) pine nuts, toasted
450	ml (16 fl oz) chicken stock
	Salt and pepper to taste

INSTRUCTIONS

To marinate the chicken breasts : In a small bowl, combine half of the olive oil, oregano, coriander, and lemon juice, and add all of the chilli powder and cumin. Stir into the chicken.

Let the chicken stand in refrigerator for 20 minutes, then drain and discard marinade.

To cook the chicken, black beans and pepper: Heat remaining olive oil in a sauté pan over high heat. Sauté chicken breast strips until cooked through.

Add beans and peppers, pine nuts and chicken stock, and heat through until peppers are slightly cooked, about 2 minutes. Season with salt and pepper. Remove from heat, stir in remaining fresh herbs and serve.

NUTRITIONAL INFORMATION:

Per Serving : 252 Calories; 7g Fat (24.6% calories from fat); 9g Protein; 40g Carbohydrate; 4g Dietary Fibre; 107mg Cholesterol; 614mg Sodium. Exchanges: 1½ Grain (Starch); ½ Lean Meat; ½ Fruit; 0 Nonfat Milk; 1 Fat, ½ Other Carbohydrates.

Mahi-Mahi Satay with Lemongrass, Brown Rice, Mange-tout and Ponzu Dipping Sauce

Serves : 4

For ponzu dipping sauce :

230	ml (8 fl oz) ponzu (Japanese citrus-base sauce available at some supermarkets, or from www.japancentre.com)
2	tbsp honey
1	tbsp chopped coriander
1	tsp finely chopped ginger
1	tsp finely chopped spring onion
1	tsp finely chopped garlic
1	tsp sambal (Asian hot sauce, available at some supermarkets)
1	tbsp sesame oil

For rice :

135	g (4¾ oz) short-grain brown rice
700	ml (1¼ pint) chicken stock
1	tbsp chopped spring onion
1	tbsp finely chopped lemongrass

For mahi-mahi satay :

115	g (4-oz) portions mahi-mahi, cut into thin strips and skewered
100	g (3½ oz) mange-tout
2	tbsp olive oil
1	tbsp soy sauce

INSTRUCTIONS

To make the ponzu dipping sauce : Combine ponzu, honey, coriander, ginger, spring onion, garlic, sambal and sesame oil.

To make the rice : In a pot, combine rice, stock, spring onion, and lemongrass. Bring to a boil, reduce heat, cover and simmer for approximately 45 minutes or until the rice is cooked.

Heat the grill or a barbecue.

To make the mahi-mahi satay : Marinate the mahi-mahi in one-quarter of the ponzu dipping sauce for 10 minutes. Place under the grill or on the barbecue and cook each side for approximately 1½ minutes.

Heat olive oil in a wok or sauté pan over high heat. When oil begins to smoke, add mange-tout and stir-fry for 2 minutes. Add soy sauce, mix in and remove from heat. Serve the skewers over rice and mange-tout with ponzu dipping sauce on the side.

NUTRITIONAL INFORMATION:

Per Serving : 374 Calories; 12g Fat (29.8% calories from fat); 25g Protein; 39g Carbohydrate; 2g Dietary Fibre; 49mg Cholesterol; 1,934mg Sodium. Exchanges: 1½ Grain (Starch); 2½ Lean Meat; 1 Vegetable; 2 Fat; ½ Other Carbohydrates.

Sherry Chicken with Brown Rice Risotto and Sautéed French Beans with Marinated Tomatoes

Serves : 4

For chicken :

35	g (1¼ oz) wholemeal flour
115	ml (4 fl oz) olive oil
100	g (3½ oz) mushrooms, sliced
2	tbsp dry sherry
350	ml (12 fl oz) chicken stock, warm
1	bay leaf
2	chicken breasts, sliced
	horizontally in 3 or 4 pieces
	Salt and pepper to taste

For haricot verts :

2	tsp olive oil
345	g (12 oz) French beans

INSTRUCTIONS

To make the sherry chicken : In a saucepan, heat 2 tablespoons olive oil and 2 tablespoons flour and cook, stirring, over medium heat until golden brown to form a 'roux'. Add mushrooms and cook for 3 minutes. Add sherry and cook for 1 minute. Add chicken stock and bay leaf and simmer for 20 minutes. Dredge chicken breast strips in remaining wholemeal flour. Heat 2 tablespoons olive oil in a sauté pan over high heat, add chicken and sauté until cooked through. Drain oil from pan. Add marsala sauce and warm through, but
do not continue to cook the chicken breast or it will become overcooked. Season with salt and pepper.

To cook the French beans : Heat olive oil in a sauté pan over medium-high heat. When oil is hot, add haricot verts and stir-fry for 3 minutes, remove from heat, and serve.

For risotto :

1 tsp olive oil
135 g (4¾ oz) short-grain brown rice
35 g (1¼ oz) onion, chopped
1 tbsp white wine
700 ml (1¼ pint) chicken stock
1 tsp extra virgin olive oil
1 tbsp grated Parmesan cheese
(optional)

For marinated tomatoes :

4 plum tomatoes,
sliced 5mm (¼ in) thick
2 tbsp balsamic vinegar
1 tsp finely chopped fresh oregano
1 tbsp fresh basil, cut into
chiffonade (thin strips)
1 tsp extra virgin olive oil
Salt and pepper to taste

To make the risotto : Heat olive oil in a saucepan over medium heat, then add onion and rice, and sweat for 2 minutes. Add white wine and cook for 1 minute, then add 230 ml (8 fl oz) chicken stock. Stir rice frequently. As liquid is absorbed and the bottom of the pan becomes visible, add another 230 ml (8 fl oz) of stock, repeating until all the stock is absorbed and the rice is tender, approximately 45 minutes. Use water if all the stock is absorbed before the rice is cooked. Drizzle with extra virgin olive oil and add Parmesan if using.

To marinate the tomatoes : Combine all ingredients.

NUTRITIONAL INFORMATION:
Per Serving : 374 Calories; 12g Fat (29.8% calories from fat); 25g Protein; 39g Carbohydrate; 2g Dietary Fibre; 49mg Cholesterol; 1,934mg Sodium. Exchanges: 1½ Grain (Starch); 2½ Lean Meat; 1 Vegetable; 2 Fat; ½ Other Carbohydrates.

Grilled Chicken Breast with Lentils, Creamless Cauliflower Gratin and Jus

Serves : 4

For marinade :

2 tbsp fresh lemon juice
2 tsp chopped fresh oregano
4 tbsp fresh basil, cut into chiffonade (thin strips)
1 clove garlic
1 tbsp extra virgin olive oil
2 boneless, skinless chicken breasts, 200–230 g (7–8 oz)

For lentils :

210 g (7½ oz) lentils (French lentils are recommended)
1 tbsp chopped carrot
1 tbsp chopped celery
1 tbsp chopped onion
1 clove garlic, finely chopped
1 tbsp chopped mushrooms
1 tbsp olive oil
2 tbsp red wine
600 ml (1 pint 1 fl oz) chicken stock
1 bay leaf
  Salt and pepper to taste

INSTRUCTIONS

Preheat the oven to 200°C/400°F/Gas mark 6. Prepare the grill or a griddle for grilling the chicken.

To make the chicken : Combine marinade ingredients, add chicken and let stand in refrigerator for 20 minutes. Drain and discard marinade. When lentils and cauliflower are almost ready cook chicken breasts under a hot grill, or in a griddle over a high heat until cooked through (approximately 10 minutes). Slice the breasts and drizzle with the jus. Serve with the lentils and cauliflower.

To make the lentils : In a saucepan over medium heat, sweat lentils, carrot, celery, onion, garlic and mushrooms in olive oil. Add red wine and cook for 2 minutes. Add chicken stock and bay leaf. Simmer until tender and liquid is absorbed, approximately 60–90 minutes. Remove bay leaf and serve.

For cauliflower gratin :

1   tbsp olive oil
½   onion, cut into julienne strips
1   head cauliflower, sliced into
      5 mm (¼-in)-thick pieces
1   clove garlic, finely chopped
1   tbsp white wine
350   ml (12 fl oz) chicken stock
1   tbsp chopped parsley
2   tsp chopped fresh thyme
1   tbsp grated Parmesan cheese (optional)
    Salt and pepper to taste

For jus :

1   tbsp chopped carrot
1   tbsp chopped celery
1   tbsp chopped onion
½   tsp finely chopped garlic
2   tsp olive oil
1   tbsp white wine
600   ml (1 pint) chicken stock
1   bay leaf .
    Salt and pepper to taste

To make the cauliflower gratin : In an oven-proof saucepan, heat olive oil over medium-low heat, add onion and cook until soft and caramelised, approximately 4 minutes. Add cauliflower and sweat for approximately 2 minutes. Add garlic and cook for approximately 30 seconds. Add wine and cook for approximately 1 minute. Add chicken stock, stir in parsley and thyme. Cover with foil and bake in 200°C/400°F/Gas mark 6 oven for 20 minutes. Remove foil, sprinkle with Parmesan (if using) and place under grill for approximately 5 minutes to brown on top.

To make the jus : Over medium heat, sweat the carrot, celery, onion and garlic in olive oil. Add white wine and cook for 2 minutes. Add chicken stock and bay leaf. Simmer for 20 minutes and strain.

NUTRITIONAL INFORMATION:

Per Serving : 556 Calories; 15g Fat (25.5% calories from fat); 50g Protein; 49g Carbohydrate; 24g Dietary Fibre; 68mg Cholesterol; 3,593mg Sodium. Exchanges: 3 Grain(Starch); 5½ Lean Meat; 1 Vegetable; 0 Fruit; 2½Fat.

PHASE IV | Sample Recipes

Breakfast | (*Phase IV*)

Recipes on the go!

- 2 (10-cm [4-inch]) pancakes
  1 tbsp syrup
  55 g (2 oz) strawberries
  230 ml (8 fl oz) semi-skimmed
       milk or orange or apple juice

- 1 mini bagel
  2 tsp jam
  1 tbsp cream cheese
  230 ml (8 fl oz) semi-skimmed
       milk or orange or apple juice

>>

- 2 slices wholemeal bread,
  toasted
  1 egg, scrambled
  5 g (⅙ oz) butter
  1 slice Cheddar cheese
  230 ml (8 fl oz) semi-skimmed
  milk
  1 medium banana

- 1 English muffin
  1 tsp syrup
  230 ml (8 fl oz) fresh orange juice
  240 g (8½ oz) low-fat yoghurt

Blueberry Buckwheat Pancakes
with Strawberry and Orange Compote

Serves : 4

For pancakes :

115	g (4 oz) buckwheat flour
30	g (1 oz) granulated sugar substitute (Splenda recommended)
2	tsp baking powder
½	tsp salt
2	large eggs, beaten
230	g (8 oz) skimmed milk
65	g (2¼ oz) blueberries
1	tbsp vegetable oil

For orange compote :

160	g (5½ oz) sliced strawberries
115	ml (4 fl oz) orange juice
1	tbsp granulated sugar substitute (Splenda recommended)

INSTRUCTIONS

To make the orange compote : Combine strawberries, orange juice and sugar substitute and cook over low heat for 25 minutes. Let stand until warm or room temperature

To make the pancakes : Sift first four ingredients together into a medium-size mixing bowl. Add eggs, milk and blueberries to dry ingredients. Do not overmix. Batter should remain slightly lumpy. Heat olive oil in nonstick pan or griddle over medium heat. Spoon 60 ml (2 fl oz) portions of pancake batter onto griddle. Cook for about 2 minutes or until edges become opaque and air bubbles on surface of pancakes begin to pop. Flip pancakes and cook for another 2 minutes.

Serve warm, drizzled with compote.

NUTRITIONAL INFORMATION:

Per Serving : 252 Calories; 7g Fat (24.6% calories from fat); 9g Protein; 40g Carbohydrate; 4g Dietary Fibre; 107mg Cholesterol; 614mg Sodium. Exchanges: 1½ Grain (Starch); ½ Lean Meat; ½ Fruit; 0 Non Fat Milk; 1 Fat; ½ Other Carbohydrates.

Banana-Stuffed Wholemeal French Toast with Mango Compote

Serves : 4

For French toast :

450	ml (16 fl oz) skimmed milk
1	large egg
1	tbsp granulated sugar substitute (Splenda recommended)
1	tsp cinnamon
2	tbsp vegetable oil
3	bananas, sliced thinly on the diagonal
8	slices wholemeal bread

For mango compote :

2	mangos, peeled, pitted and chopped
3	tbsp granulated sugar substitute (Splenda recommended)

INSTRUCTIONS

To make the mango compote : Combine mangos and sugar substitute and cook over low heat for 20 minutes. Let stand until warm or room temperature.

To make the French toast : Mix milk, egg, sugar substitute and cinnamon. Heat olive oil in nonstick pan or griddle over medium heat. Distribute banana slices on four slices of bread, then gently press remaining four slices of bread on top of each bottom slice. Dip bread in milk and egg mixture, and cook over medium heat for about 3 minutes per side, or until golden.

Spoon mango compote over each serving.

NUTRITIONAL INFORMATION:

Per Serving : 399 Calories; 11g Fat (23.9% calories from fat); 12g Protein; 67g Carbohydrate; 7g Dietary Fibre; 55mg Cholesterol; 402mg Sodium. Exchanges: 1½ Grain (Starch); 0 Lean Meat; 2 Fruit; ½ Skimmed Milk; 2 Fat; ½ Other Carbohydrates.

Egg White Omelette with Low-Fat Cheddar Cheese and Fresh Herbs

Serves : 4

18	egg whites
1	tsp finely chopped fresh thyme
1	tsp finely chopped fresh parsley
1	tsp finely chopped fresh chives
	Salt and pepper to taste
2	tbsp olive oil
180	g (6½ oz) grated low-fat Cheddar cheese
80	g (2¾ oz) sliced strawberries

INSTRUCTIONS

Whisk together egg whites, herbs, salt and pepper.

In a non-stick omelette pan, heat one-quarter of the oil and pour in one-quarter of the egg white mixture.

Cook until set, stirring constantly with a rubber spatula.

Stir in one-quarter of the cheese, fold omelette over and serve with strawberries.

Repeat for 3 more omelettes.

NUTRITIONAL INFORMATION:

Per Serving : 215 Calories; 10g Fat (42.3% calories from fat); 26g Protein; 4g Carbohydrate; 1g Dietary Fibre; 9mg Cholesterol; 506mg Sodium. Exchanges: 0 Grain (Starch); 3½ Lean Meat; 0 Vegetable; 0 Fruit; 1½ Fat.

Dinner | (*Phase IV*)

Ahi Fish Tacos with Roasted Poblano Guacamole

Serves : 4

4   whole wheat tortillas

For tuna :

¼   tsp chilli powder
¼   tsp cumin
¼   tsp dried oregano
   Salt and pepper to taste
¼   tsp cayenne pepper
¼   tsp cinnamon
285   g (10 oz) tuna steak, sliced 1-cm (½-in)-thick
1   tbsp olive oil
1   tbsp rice wine vinegar
1   tbsp lemon juice
2   tbsp Tabasco
45   g (1½ oz), shredded iceberg lettuce
1   red pepper, cut into julienne strips
½   red onion, cut into julienne strips
3   tbs (rounded) chopped fresh coriander

INSTRUCTIONS

To make the tuna : Combine chilli powder, cumin, dried oregano, salt, pepper, cayenne pepper and cinnamon, and sprinkle on fish to season. In a sauté pan, heat oil over high heat. Sear tuna over very high heat (tuna should remain slightly pink in centre). Combine vinegar, lemon juice and Tabasco and toss with lettuce, pepper, red onion and coriander.

For guacamole :

1 small chilli pepper, roasted,
    peeled and chopped
1 small avocado, peeled and
    chopped
1 tsp lemon juice
1 clove garlic, finely chopped
1 tbsp chopped plum
    tomato
1 tbsp chopped red onion
1 tbsp finely chopped coriander
   Salt and pepper to taste

To make the guacamole : Combine chilli pepper, avocado, lemon juice, garlic, tomato, red onion, coriander, salt and pepper and blend well.

To assemble : Place fish and vegetable mixture into tortillas, roll up and cut tortillas in half.

Serve two halves per serving. Garnish with guacamole.

NUTRITIONAL INFORMATION:

Per Serving : 384 Calories; 17g Fat (39.5% calories from fat); 23g Protein; 37g Carbohydrate; 5g Dietary Fibre; 27mg Cholesterol; 695mg Sodium. Exchanges: 0 Grain (Starch); 2½ Lean Meat; 1 Vegetable; 0 Fruit; 2 Fat; 0 Other Carbohydrates.

Roasted Chicken Breast with Brown Saffron Risotto, Oven-Dried Tomatoes and Basil/Mint Jus

Serves : 4

For chicken breast :

2	boneless and skinless chicken breasts, 200–230 g (7–8 oz) each
	Salt and pepper to taste

For basil/mint jus :

1	tbsp chopped carrot
1	tbsp chopped celery
1	tbsp chopped onion
½	tsp finely chopped garlic
2	tsp olive oil
1	tbsp white wine
600	ml (1 pint) chicken stock
2	sprigs fresh basil
2	sprigs fresh mint
1	bay leaf
	Salt and pepper to taste

For oven-dried tomatoes :

16	plum tomatoes, quartered (see shortcut substitution below)
1	tbsp olive oil

INSTRUCTIONS

Preheat oven to 200°C/400°F/Gas mark 6.

To roast the chicken breasts : Roast breasts in a 200°C/400°F/Gas mark 6 oven until done, approximately 10 minutes. Let cool and slice into strips.

To make the basil/mint jus : Over medium heat, sweat carrot, celery, onion and garlic in olive oil. Add white wine and cook for 2 minutes. Add chicken stock, basil, mint and bay leaf. Simmer for 20 minutes. Season with salt and pepper. Strain.

To make the oven-dried tomatoes : Preheat oven to 110°C/225°F/Gas mark ¼. Drizzle tomatoes with olive oil. Place in oven for 4 hours and remove. Let cool.
(Note substitution: You can use sun-dried tomatoes, simmered in water for 10 minutes and drained, then tossed with olive oil.)

For risotto :

2	tsp olive oil
2	tbsp yellow onion, peeled and chopped
400	g (14 oz) short-grain brown rice
1	tbsp white wine
1.6	litres (2 pints 16 oz) chicken stock, hot
1	tbsp saffron
1	tsp p olive oil
	Salt and pepper to taste
1	tbsp grated Parmesan cheese (optional)

To make the risotto : (Tip: Keep chicken stock simmering in a separate pot next to the risotto.) Heat olive oil in saucepan, over medium heat, add onion and rice, and sweat for 2 minutes. Add white wine and cook for 1 minute, then add 1 cup (approx 8 fl oz) chicken stock and saffron. Stir rice frequently. As liquid is absorbed and the bottom of the pan is visible, add another cup of stock, repeating until all stock is absorbed, approximately 45 minutes. Drizzle with extra virgin olive oil and add Parmesan if using.

To serve : Spoon risotto into bowls and add tomatoes and chicken.

NUTRITIONAL INFORMATION:

Per Serving : 721 Calories; 15g Fat (19.6% calories from fat); 41g Protein; 99g Carbohydrate; 7g Dietary Fibre; 68mg Cholesterol; 5228mg Sodium. Exchanges: 5 Grain (Starch); 4 Lean Meat; 4½ Vegetable; 2 Fat.

SNACKS:

CHOOSE ONLY ONE SNACK FOR THE ALLOTTED SNACK PERIOD IN YOUR EATING SCHEDULE. CHOOSE THE SNACK THAT FITS THE PHASE YOU'RE CURRENTLY IN.

- 80 g (2¾ oz) cup plain low-fat yoghurt dip and 240 g (8½ oz) raw vegetables

- Cashew nuts (10)

- 2 digestive biscuits and 2 tsp reduced-sugar jam

- 1 low-fat cereal bar

- 15 grapes and 115 ml (4 fl oz) of semi-skimmed milk

- 115 g (4 oz) of plain low-fat yoghurt

- 2 tbsp raisins and 10 peanuts

- 1 small brownie

- 2 ginger snap biscuits and 15 g (½ oz) Cheddar cheese

- baby carrots

- 2 chocolate chip cookies, small

- Tortilla chips, (8–10)

- 40 g licorice

- Almonds (10–14)

- 1 small pot low-fat raspberry mousse

- 3 rich tea biscuits

- Popcorn, air-popped (12 g, no butter!)

- 2 rice cakes topped with 1 tsp peanut butter

- 1 cup unsweetened applesauce

- Water biscuits, small (7)

- 1 medium banana, frozen

- 8 halves dried apricots and 115 ml (4 fl oz) skimmed milk

- Sunflower seeds (2 tbsp)

- 1 small pot low-fat chocolate mousse

- Melba toast (4 slices)

- 6 water biscuits topped with 2 tsp reduced-sugar jam

DR. IAN'S TIP : Skip the power bars. They are convenient and attractively packaged, but are high in calories and sugar.

APPENDICES

Body Mass Index Chart

Fibre Content of Foods

How to Read a Food Label

Caloric Expenditure During Various Activities

BODY MASS INDEX (*BMI*)

Height	18	19	20	21	22	23	24	25	26	27	28	29	30	31	32	33	34	35	36	37	38	39	40
										Body Weight (pounds)													
4'10" 147cm	86	91	96	100	105	110	115	119	124	129	134	138	143	148	153	158	162	167	172	177	181	186	191
4'11" 150cm	89	94	99	104	109	114	119	124	128	133	138	143	148	153	158	163	168	173	178	183	188	193	198
5'0" 152cm	92	97	102	107	112	118	123	128	133	138	143	148	153	158	163	168	174	179	184	189	194	199	204
5'1" 155cm	95	100	106	111	116	122	127	132	137	143	148	153	158	164	169	174	180	185	190	195	201	206	211
5'2" 157cm	98	104	109	115	120	126	131	136	142	147	153	158	164	169	175	180	186	191	196	202	207	213	218
5'3" 160cm	102	107	113	118	124	130	135	141	146	152	158	163	169	175	180	186	191	197	203	208	214	220	225
5'4" 163cm	105	110	116	122	128	134	140	145	151	157	163	169	174	180	186	192	197	204	209	215	221	227	232
5'5" 165cm	108	114	120	126	132	138	144	150	156	162	168	174	180	186	192	198	204	210	216	222	228	234	240
5'6" 168cm	112	118	124	130	136	142	148	155	161	167	173	179	186	192	198	204	210	216	223	229	235	241	247
5'7" 170cm	115	121	127	134	140	146	153	159	166	172	178	185	191	198	204	211	217	223	230	236	242	249	255
5'8" 173cm	118	125	131	138	144	151	158	165	171	177	184	190	197	203	210	216	223	230	236	243	249	256	262
5'9" 175cm	122	128	135	142	149	155	162	169	176	182	189	196	203	209	216	223	230	236	243	250	257	263	270
5'10" 178cm	126	132	139	146	153	160	167	174	181	188	195	202	209	216	222	229	236	243	250	257	264	271	278
5'11" 180cm	129	136	143	150	157	165	172	179	186	193	200	208	215	222	229	236	243	250	257	265	272	279	286
6'0" 183cm	132	140	147	154	162	169	177	184	191	199	206	213	221	228	235	242	250	258	265	272	279	287	294
6'1" 185cm	136	144	151	159	166	174	182	189	197	204	212	219	227	235	242	250	257	265	272	280	288	295	302
6'2" 188cm	141	148	155	163	171	179	186	194	202	210	218	225	233	241	249	256	264	272	280	287	295	303	311
6'3" 190cm	144	152	160	168	176	184	192	200	208	216	224	232	240	248	256	264	272	279	287	295	303	311	319
6'4" 193cm	148	156	164	172	180	189	197	205	213	221	230	238	246	254	263	271	279	287	295	304	312	320	328
6'5" 196cm	151	160	168	176	185	193	202	210	218	227	235	244	252	261	269	277	286	294	303	311	319	328	336
6'6" 198cm	155	164	172	181	190	198	207	216	224	233	241	250	259	267	276	284	293	302	310	319	328	336	345

UNDERWEIGHT	HEALTHY WEIGHT	OVERWEIGHT	OBESE
(<18.5)	(18.5–24.9)	(25–29.9)	(≥30)

To use this chart you will first need to calculate your weight in pounds. This is easiest if you start with kilograms: simply multiply the kilos by 2.2. If you prefer to use stone, multiply the number of stone by 14 and add this figure and pounds left over. Next, find your height in centimetres or feet and inches. Finally look across the row until you find the number that is closest to your weight. The number at the top of that column identifies your BMI.

Source: From A. Must, G. E. Dallal, and W. H. Dietz, "Reference Data for Obesity: 85th and 95th Percentiles of Body Mass Index (wt/ht²) and Triceps Skinfold Thickness." *American Journal of Clinical Nutrition 53* (1991): 839–846. Adapted with permission by the *American Journal of Clinical Nutrition*, © *American Journal of Clinical Nutrition*, American Society fo Clinical Nutrition.

FIBRE CONTENT OF FOODS

To consume more fibre, eat more whole fruits and vegetables, whole grains and beans. Nuts are also rich in fibre, but they are energy dense, so eat them in small amounts. Use the following list to guide your food choices. It is adapted from research conducted by the Tufts University School of Medicine in Boston, U.S.A. and published in the *Tufts Health & Nutrition Letter*.

FRUITS*	GRAMS OF FIBRE
Apple (with skin)	4
Banana	3
Blueberries, 65 g (2¼ oz)	2
Cantaloupe, 140 g (5 oz), chopped	1
Dates, 20 g (⅔ oz) dry, chopped	2
Grapefruit, ½	2
Grapes, 140 g (5 oz)	2
Nectarine (with skin)	2
Orange	3
Peach (with skin)	2
Pear (with skin)	4
Plum (with skin)	1
Prunes (dried), 10	2
Raisins, 20 g (⅔ oz)	1
Raspberries, 55 g (2 oz)	4
Strawberries, 55 g (2 oz)	2
Watermelon, 140 g (5 oz), chopped	1

VEGETABLES†	GRAMS OF FIBRE
Broccoli, 55 g (2 oz), chopped	2
Broccoli, 45 g (1½ oz) chopped	1

*All values are for 1 medium-size fruit unless otherwise indicated.

†All values are for raw, uncooked vegetables unless otherwise indicated.

Brussels sprouts, ½ cup cooked	3
Carrot, 1 medium	2
Carrots, 55g (2 oz), sliced, cooked	3
Cauliflower, 55g (2 oz), cooked	2
Celery, 1 stick	1
Chips, 1 small serving (70 g [2½ oz])	2
Cucumber, 55g (2 oz), sliced	0.5
Green beans 45 g (1½ oz), cooked (frozen)	2
Iceberg lettuce 45 g (1½ oz), shredded	1
Peas, 80 g (2¾ oz), cooked (frozen)	4
Peppers, 65 g (2¼ oz), chopped	1
Potato, baked, with skin	5
Potato, baked, without skin	2
Potato, 115 g (4 oz), mashed	2
Romaine/cos lettuce, 30 g (1 oz), shredded	1
Spinach, 55 g (2 oz), chopped	1
Spinach, 115 g (4 oz), cooked (frozen)	3
Sweetcorn, 70 g (2½ oz)	2
Sweet potato, baked with skin	3
Tomato, 1 medium	1

GRAINS, PULSES* (BEANS, CHICKPEAS, LENTILS, BROAD BEANS), AND NUTS	GRAMS OF FIBRE
Black beans, 80 g (2¾ oz)	8
Bread, 1 slice, white	1
Bread, 1 slice, wholemeal	2
Broad beans, 55 g (2 oz)	6

*Values are for canned or cooked beans.

(Grains, Pulses and Nuts, continued)	GRAMS OF FIBRE
Chickpeas, 80 g (2¾ oz)	5
Kidney beans, 65 g (2¼ oz)	7
Lentils, 70 g (2½ oz)	8
Oatmeal, 160 g (5½ oz), cooked	4
Pasta, 90 g (3 oz), cooked	1
Peanuts, 100 g (3½ oz)	6
Peanut butter, 2 tablespoons, chunky	2
Popcorn, 30 g (1 oz), air-popped	2
Rice, 160 g (5½ oz), cooked, white	1
Rice, 160 g (5½ oz), cooked, brown	2
Sesame seeds, 2 tablespoons	1
Sunflower seeds, 20 g (⅔ oz)	2
Tortilla chips, 45 g (1½ oz)	1
Walnuts, 35 g (1¼ oz), chopped	2
Wheat germ, 10 g (⅓ oz)	4

HOW TO READ A FOOD LABEL

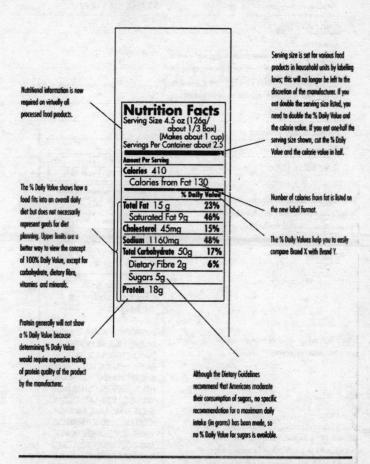

Nutritional information is now required on virtually all processed food products.

The % Daily Value shows how a food fits into an overall daily diet but does not necessarily represent goals for diet planning. Upper limits are a better way to view the concept of 100% Daily Value, except for carbohydrate, dietary fibre, vitamins and minerals.

Protein generally will not show a % Daily Value because determining % Daily Value would require expensive testing of protein quality of the product by the manufacturer.

Serving size is set for various food products in household units by labelling laws; this will no longer be left to the discretion of the manufacturer. If you eat double the serving size listed, you need to double the % Daily Value and the calorie value. If you eat one-half the serving size shown, cut the % Daily Value and the calorie value in half.

Number of calories from fat is listed on the new label format.

The % Daily Values help you to easily compare Brand X with Brand Y.

Although the Dietary Guidelines recommend that Americans moderate their consumption of sugars, no specific recommendation for a maximum daily intake (in grams) has been made, so no % Daily Value for sugars is available.

Nutrition Facts
Serving Size 4.5 oz (126g/
about 1/3 Box)
(Makes about 1 cup)
Servings Per Container about 2.5

Amount Per Serving

Calories 410

Calories from Fat 130

	% Daily Value*
Total Fat 15 g	23%
Saturated Fat 9g	46%
Cholesterol 45mg	15%
Sodium 1160mg	48%
Total Carbohydrate 50g	17%
Dietary Fibre 2g	6%
Sugars 5g	
Protein 18g	

The Nutrition Facts panel on a current food label. The box is broken into two parts: A is the top, and B is the bottom. The % Daily Value listed on the label is the percentage of the generally accepted amount of a nutrient needed daily that is present in 1 serving of the product. You can use the % Daily Values to compare your diet with current nutrition recommendations for certain diet components. Let's consider dietary fibre. Assume that you consume 2,000 kcal. per day, which is the energy intake corresponding to the % Daily Values listed on labels. If the total % Daily Value for dietary fibre in all the foods you eat in one day adds up to 100%, your diet meets the recommendations for dietary fibre.

150

Many vitamin and mineral amounts no longer need to be listed on the nutrition label. Only Vitamin A, Vitamin C, calcium, and iron remain. The interest in or risk of deficiencies of the other vitamins and minerals is deemed too low to warrant inclusion.

Some % Daily Value standards, such as grams of total fat, increase as energy intake increases. The % Daily Values on the label are based on a 2,000-kcal. diet. This is important to note if you don't consume at least 2,000 kcal. per day.

Labels on larger packages may list the number of calories per gram of fat, carbohydrate and protein.

Ingredients, listed in descending order by weight, will appear here or in another place on the package. The sources of some ingredients, such as certain flavourings, will be stated by name to help people better identify ingredients that they avoid for health, religious or other reasons.

Vitamin A 10% • Vitamin C 0%
Calcium 30% • Iron 15%

Percent Daily Values are based on a 2,000 calorie diet. Your daily values may be higher or lower depending on your calorie needs:

	Calories:	2,000	2,500
Total Fat	Less than	65g	80g
Sat Fat	Less than	20g	25g
Cholest	Less than	300mg	300mg
Sodium	Less than	2,400mg	2,400mg
Total Carb		300g	375g
Fiber		25g	30g

Calories per gram:
Fat 9 • Carbohydrate 4 • Protein 4

INGREDIENTS: WATER, ENRICHED MACARONI (ENRICHED FLOUR [NIACIN, FERROUS SULFATE (IRON), THIAMINE MONONITRATE AND RIBOFLAVIN], EGG WHITE), FLOUR, CHEDDAR CHEESE (MILK, CHEESE CULTURE, SALT, ENZYME), SPICES, MARGARINE (PARTIALLY HYDROGENATED SOYBEAN OIL, WATER, SOY LECITHIN, MONO- AND DIGLYCERIDES, BETA CARO-TENE FOR COLOR, VITAMIN A PALMITATE), AND MALTODEXTRIN.

Source: Wardlaw, Gordon M., *Contemporary Nutrition*, 4th ed. (New York: McGraw Hill Companies, Inc., 2000).

CALORIC EXPENDITURE
DURING VARIOUS ACTIVITIES

ACTIVITY	CAL/MIN*
Sleeping	1.2
Resting in bed	1.3
Sitting, normally	1.3
Sitting, reading	1.3
Lying, quietly	1.3
Sitting, eating	1.5
Sitting, playing cards	1.5
Standing, normally	1.5
Classwork, lecture (listening)	1.7
Conversing	1.0
Personal grooming	2.0
Sitting, writing	2.6
Standing, light activity	2.6
Washing and dressing	2.6
Washing and shaving	2.6
Driving a car	2.8
Washing clothes	3.1
Walking indoors	3.1
Shining shoes	3.2
Making bed	3.4
Dressing	3.4
Showering	3.4
Riding motorcycle	3.4

*Depends on efficiency and body size. Add 10 percent for each 6.8 Kilos (15 lb) over 150; subtract 10 percent for each 6.8 Kilos (15 lb) under 150.

ACTIVITY	CAL/MIN
Metalworking	3.5
House painting	3.5
Cleaning windows	3.7
Carpentry	3.8
Farming chores	3.8
Sweeping floors	3.9
Plastering walls	4.1
Repairing trucks and automobiles	4.2
Ironing clothes	4.2
Farming, planting, hoeing, raking	4.7
Mixing cement	4.7
Mopping floors	4.9
Repaving roads	5.0
Gardening, weeding	5.6
Stacking timber	5.8
Sawing with chain saw	6.2
Working with stone, masonry	6.3
Working with pick and shovel	6.7
Farming, haying, ploughing with horse	6.7
Shovelling (miners)	6.8
Shovelling snow	7.5
Walking down stairs	7.1
Chopping wood	7.5
Sawing with crosscut saw	7.5–10.5
Tree felling (axe)	8.4–12.7
Gardening, digging	8.6
Walking up stairs	10.0–18.0
Playing pool or billiards	1.8
Canoeing, 2.5 mph-4.0 mph	3.0–7.0

ACTIVITY	CAL/MIN
Playing volleyball, recreational to competitive	3.5–8.0
Golfing, foursome to twosome	3.7–5.0
Pitching horseshoes	3.8
Playing baseball (except pitcher)	4.7
Playing Ping-Pong or table tennis	4.9–7.0
Practicing calisthenics	5.0
Rowing, pleasure to vigorous	5.0–15.0
Cycling, easy to hard	5.0–15.0
Skating, recreational to vigorous	5.0–15.0
Practising archery	5.2
Playing badminton, recreational to competitive	5.2–10.0
Playing basketball, half or full court (more for fast break)	6.0–9.0
Bowling (while active)	7.0
Playing tennis, recreational to competitive	7.0–11.0
Waterskiing	8.0
Playing soccer	9.0
Snowshoeing (2.5 mph)	9.0
Slide board	9.0–13.0
Playing handball or squash	10.0
Mountain climbing	10.0–15.0
Skipping rope	10.0–15.0
Practicing judo or karate	13.0
Playing American football (while active)	13.3
Wrestling	14.4
Skiing	
Moderate to steep	8.0–20.0

ACTIVITY	CAL/MIN
Downhill racing	16.5
Cross-country; 3–10 mph	9.0–20.0
Swimming	
Leisurely	6.0
Crawl, 25-50 yd/min.	6.0–12.5
Butterfly, 50 yd/min.	14.0
Backstroke, 25-50 yd/min.	6.0–12.5
Breaststroke, 25-50 yd/min.	6.0–12.5
Sidestroke, 40 yd/min.	11.0
Dancing	
Modern, moderate to vigorous	4.2–5.7
Ballroom, waltz to rumba	5.7–7.0
Square	77
Walking	
Road or field (3.5 mph)	5.6–7.0
Snow, hard to soft (2.5–3.5 mph)	10.0–20.0
Uphill, 15 percent grade (3.5mph)	8.0–15.0
Downhill, 5-10 percent grade(2.5 mph)	3.5–3.7
15-20 percent grade (2.5 mph)	3.7–4.3
Hiking, 40-lb. pack (3.0 mph)	6.8
Running	
12-min. mile (5 mph)	10.0
8-min. mile (7.5 mph)	15.0
6-min. mile (10 mph)	20.0
5-min. mile (12 mph)	25.0

Source: Adapted from Sharkey, Brian J., PhD., *Fitness and Health*, 4th ed. (Champaign: Human Kinetics, 1997).

BIBLIOGRAPHY

Books

Atkins, Robert C., M.D., *Dr. Atkin's Diet Revolution* (New York: Bantam, 1972).

Brody, Tom, *Nutritional Biochemistry*, 2nd ed (Academic Press, 1999).

Cooper, Kenneth H., M.D., M.PH., *The Aerobics Program for Total Well-Being* (New York. Bantam Books, 1982)

Hensrud, Donald D., M.D., *Mayo Clinic on Healthy Weight* (New York: Kensington Publishing Corporation, 2000).

Katch, Frank I., and McArdle, William D., *Introduction to Nutrition, Exercise, and Health*, 4th ed. (Baltimore: Lippincott Williams and Wilkins, 1988).

Mathews, Christopher K., and van Holde, K. E., *Biochemistry* (Redwood City, Calif.: Benjamin/Cummings Publishing Company, 1990).

McArdle, William D., Katch, Frank I., and Katch, Victor L., *Exercise Physiology: Energy, Nutrition, and Human Performance*, 4th ed. (New York: Lippincott Williams and Wilkins, 1996).

Paulsen, Barbara, *The Diet Advisor* (New York: Time-Life Books, 2000).

Rolls, Barbara, Ph.D., and Barnett, Robert, *Volumetrics Weight-Control Plan* (New York: HarperCollins, 2000).

Sears, Barry, Ph.D., *The Zone* (New York: HarperCollins, 1995).

Sharkey, Brian J., PhD., *Fitness and Health*, 4th ed. (Champaign: Human Kinetics, 1997).

Sizer, Frances, and Whitney, Eleanor, *Nutrition: Concepts and Controversies*, 8th ed. (Stamford: Wadsworth/Thomson Learning, 2000).

Steward, H. Leighton, Bethea, Morrison C., Nadrews, Sam S., Brennan, Ralph O., and Balart, Luis A. , *Sugar Busters!: Cut Sugar to Trim Fat* (New York: Ballantine, 1998).

Tarnower, Herman, and Baker, Samm Sinclair *Complete Scarsdale Medical Diet*

Plus Dr. Tarnower's Lifetime Keep-Slim Program (New York: Bantam Books, 1995).

Wardlaw, Gordon M., *Contemporary Nutrition: Issues and Insights,* 4th ed. (New York: The McGraw-Hill Companies, Inc., 2000).

Studies/Articles

The American Dietetics' Association Food and Nutrition Guide.

Willett, W.C., Dietz, W. H., and Colditz, G. A., "Guidelines for Healthy Weight," *New England Journal of Medicine* 341 (1999): 427–34.

National Institutes of Health, "Clinical Guidelines on the Identification, Evaluation, and Treatment of Overweight and Obesity in Adults" (September 1998).

U.S. Department of Health and Human Services, "Physical Activity and Health: A Report of the Surgeon General" (Atlanta, GA.: Centers for Disease Control and Prevention, National Center for Chronic Disease Prevention and Health Promotion, 1996).

Paffenbarger, R. S., Hyde, R. T., Wing, A. L., et al., "The Association of Changes in Physical-Activity Level and Other Lifestyle Characteristics with Mortality Among Men," *New England Journal of Medicine* 328, no. 8 (1993): 538–45.

Sherman, S. E., D'Agostino, R. B., Cobb, J. L., et al., "Physical Activity and Mortality in Women in the Framingham Heart Study," *American Heart Journal* 128, no. 5 (1994): 879–84.

Pate, R. R., Pratt, M., Blair, S. N., et al. "Physical Activity and Public Health: A Recommendation from the Centers for Disease Control and Prevention and the American College of Sports Medicine," *Journal of the American Medical Association* 273, no. 5 (1995): 402–407.

USDA and U.S. Department of Health and Human Services, *Dietary Guidelines for Americans,* 5th ed. (USDA Home and Garden Bulletin No. 232. Washington, D.C.: USDA, 2000).

USDA, *The Food Guide Pyramid* (USDA Home and Garden Bulletin No. 252. Washington, D.C.: USDA, 1992).

Flegal, K. M., Carroll, M.D., Kuczmarski, R. J., et al, "Overweight and Obesity in the United States: Prevalence and Trends, 1960–1994," *International Journal of Obesity* 22, no. 1 (1998): 39–47.

NIH, "Clinical Guideline on the Identification, Evaluation and Treatment of Overweight and Obesity in Adults—The Evidence Report," *Obesity Research* 6 (suppl. 2, 1998): 51S–209S.

PHS, *The Surgeon General's Report on Nutrition and Health* (DHHS Pub. No. [PHS] 88050210, Washington, D.C.: HHS, 1988).

INDEX

ABOUT THE AUTHOR

Dr. Ian Smith is a medical contributor to ABC's nationally syndicated *The View*, a medical columnist for *Men's Health* magazine, and the medical/diet expert on VH1's *Celebrity Fit Club*. Dr. Smith is also the host of the nationally syndicated radio show *Healthwise* on American Urban Radio Networks. He was formerly a medical correspondent for NBC News and for NewsChannel 4, where he filed reports for NBC's *Nightly News* and the *Today* show as well as WNBC's news broadcasts. He has written for a variety of publications including *Time, Newsweek* and the New York *Daily News*, and has been featured in *People, Essence, Ebony, Cosmopolitan* and *University of Chicago Medicine on the Midway*.

Dr. Smith graduated from Harvard College with an AB and received a master's in science education from Columbia University. He attended Dartmouth Medical School and completed the last two years of his medical education at the University of Chicago Pritzker School of Medicine.

Dr. Smith is also the author of three other books: *The Blackbird Papers: A Novel* (2005 BCALA fiction Honor Book Award winner), *Dr. Ian Smith's Guide to Medical Websites* and *The Take-Control Diet*.